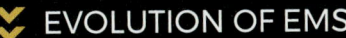
COVID-19 GUIDANCE

FOR EMS PROVIDERS

COVID-19 GUIDANCE
FOR EMS PROVIDERS

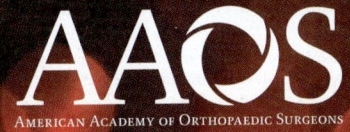

Medical Editor:
Andrew N. Pollak, MD, FAAOS

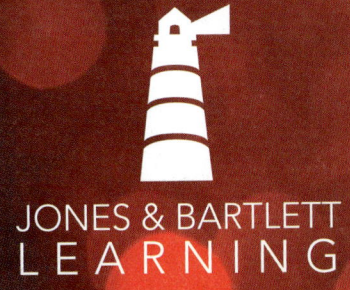

World Headquarters
Jones & Bartlett Learning
5 Wall Street
Burlington, MA 01803
978-443-5000
info@jblearning.com
www.jblearning.com
www.psglearning.com

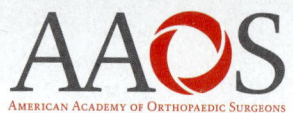

Substantial discounts on bulk quantities of Jones & Bartlett Learning publications are available to corporations, professional associations, and other qualified organizations. For details and specific discount information, contact the special sales department at Jones & Bartlett Learning via the above contact information or send an email to specialsales@jblearning.com.

Jones & Bartlett Learning books and products are available through most bookstores and online booksellers. To contact the Jones & Bartlett Learning Public Safety Group directly, call 800-832-0034, fax 978-443-8000, or visit our website, www.psglearning.com.

22941-7

Production Credits
VP, Product Development: Christine Emerton
Director, Product Management: Jonathan Epstein
Director, Content Management: Donna Gridley
Product Manager: Carly Mahoney
Content Strategist: Tiffany Sliter
Content Strategist: MT Cozzola
Content Coordinator: Paula Gregory
Director of Marketing Operations: Brian Rooney
VP, Sales: Phil Charland
Project Manager: Kristen Rogers
Project Specialist: Meghan McDonagh

Senior Digital Project Specialist: Angela Dooley
Content Services Manager: Colleen Lamy
VP, Manufacturing and Inventory Control: Therese Connell
Composition: S4Carlisle Publishing Services
Cover Design: Scott Moden
Text Design: Scott Moden
Senior Media Development Editor: Troy Liston
Rights & Permissions Manager: John Rusk
Rights Specialist: Rebecca Damon
Cover Image (Title Page): © KaiMook Studio 99/Shutterstock
Printing and Binding: LSC Communications

Library of Congress Cataloging-in-Publication Data
Library of Congress Cataloging-in-Publication Data unavailable at time of printing.

LCCN: 2020950415

6048

Printed in the United States of America
24 23 22 21 20   10 9 8 7 6 5 4 3 2 1

Table of Contents

Preface

As an EMS provider, staying safe through the evolving COVID-19 pandemic presents distinct challenges. That's why the Public Safety Group, in partnership with the American Academy of Orthopaedic Surgeons, is pleased to introduce *Evolution of EMS: COVID-19 Guidance for EMS Providers*. This resource offers strategies and insights designed specifically for you.

 Evolution of EMS: COVID-19 Guidance for EMS Providers describes the SARS-CoV-2 virus, the disease it causes in people (COVID-19), prevention tactics, vaccine development, treatment, and public health implications, particularly as they affect providers working in the field. It is not designed to cover everything there is to know about COVID-19, but rather to brief you on key issues and considerations. *Evolution of EMS: COVID-19 Guidance for EMS Providers* also offers references for learning more and staying up to date. The goal: empowering you to protect yourself, your coworkers, and the people you serve more efficiently and effectively.

Acknowledgments

The Jones & Bartlett Learning Public Safety Group and the American Academy of Orthopaedic Surgeons would like to thank the contributors and reviewers of *Evolution of EMS: COVID-19 Guidance for EMS Providers*.

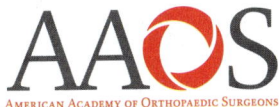

Medical Editor

Andrew N. Pollak, MD, FAAOS
Medical Director Baltimore County Fire Department
The James Lawrence Kernan Professor and Chairman
Department of Orthopaedics
University of Maryland School of Medicine
Senior Vice President for Clinical Transformation and
    Chief of Orthopaedics
University of Maryland Medical System
Special Deputy US Marshal
Baltimore, Maryland

Contributors

Stephanie Ashford, EdS, MEd, CCP-C
Quality and Patient Safety Coordinator
St. Charles County Ambulance District
St. Peters, Missouri

Andrew Bartkus, JD, MSN, RN, NRP, CEN, CCRN, CFRN, Esq.
Emergency Department Director
Sandoval Regional Medical Center
Rio Rancho, New Mexico

Dennis Edgerly, MEd, EMTP
Director EMS Academy
Arapahoe Community College
Littleton, Colorado

Michael A. Kaduce, MPS, NRP
EMT Program Director
UCLA Center for Prehospital Care
Los Angeles, California

Reviewers

Barbara Aehlert, MSEd, RN
Southwest EMS Education, Inc.
Burnet, Texas

James Brasiel, MD
Ready Enterprises
Concord, California

Rommie L. Duckworth, BS, LP
New England Center for Rescue & Emergency Medicine
Sherman, Connecticut

Kelly Kohler, MS, Paramedic, CCP-C, CHSE, NCEE
Touro College of Osteopathic Medicine
Middletown, New York

Guy Peifer
Yonkers Fire Department
Yonkers, New York

Stephen Rahm, NRP
Centre for Emergency Health Sciences
Spring Branch, Texas

Christopher Touzeau, MS, FNP-C, NRP
Montgomery County Fire Rescue Training Academy
Montgomery Village, Maryland

PART 1
Understanding COVID-19 Infection and Illness

Effective protocols and precautions for working with patients who have COVID-19 start with a basic understanding of severe acute respiratory syndrome coronavirus 2, or SARS-CoV-2, the virus that causes the COVID-19 disease.

Coronaviruses: An Overview

SARS-CoV-2 is a type of coronavirus. As such, it shares some important characteristics with other coronaviruses.

All viruses are microscopic in size, several times smaller than bacteria. They contain either RNA or DNA but cannot reproduce without a host. A virus spreads by invading host cells and then using the structure of the host's cells to replicate. Thus, viruses have been referred to as intracellular parasites. Treatment of viral illnesses is tricky because viruses can gain access to the inside of the host's cells and essentially hide. Viruses exist throughout nature and across all known species. Some viruses infect only nonhuman species, whereas others can infect both nonhumans and humans.

Coronaviruses contain RNA and belong to the virus family Coronaviridae, falling within one of two broad subcategories: Coronavirinae and Torovirinae. Both groups contain viruses found in nonhumans, but only those in the Coronavirinae group are known to cause disease in humans.[1]

The name coronavirus comes from the Latin word *corona*, which means crown. It refers to the distinctive, crown-like appearance of the projections located on the protective envelope surrounding the virus's genetic material (**FIGURE 1-1**). These projections are what enable the virus to attach to the host's cells.

Where Coronaviruses Come From

Although the exact origin of coronaviruses is not known, the first incidence of this type of virus was identified in chickens in the 1930s. In the 1960s, a

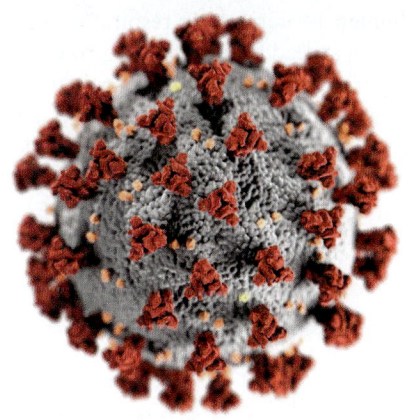

FIGURE 1-1 An illustration of a coronavirus.
Courtesy of CDC/Alissa Eckert, MSMI; Dan Higgins, MAMS.

human coronavirus, distinct from more common rhinoviruses, was identified as a cause of the common cold in approximately 2% to 10% of patients experiencing cold-like symptoms.[2]

Human coronaviruses were not considered a serious concern to humans until 2003, when a coronavirus responsible for causing severe acute respiratory syndrome (SARS) became evident. Originally found in nonhuman animals, including bats and civet cats (a species native to tropical Asia and Africa), the virus adapted and spread to humans. SARS affects the upper and lower respiratory systems and causes coughing, sneezing, runny nose, and pneumonia.

In 2003, approximately 8,000 probable SARS cases were reported to the World Health Organization (WHO), with 774 related deaths, a case fatality rate of 9.6%. WHO declared a pandemic, indicating the virus had spread rapidly throughout multiple countries. Governments responded with travel limitations and other precautions, and the spread of SARS was halted. Currently, there is no known human-to-human spread of SARS-CoV, but reemergence of the virus remains possible in the future from nonhuman reservoirs.[3]

Middle East Respiratory Syndrome (MERS-CoV) is another example of a coronavirus. It first presented in 2012 in Saudi Arabia. Experts believe the virus originated in nonhuman hosts (camels) and transferred to humans. The virus transfers from human to human via respiratory secretions and is often spread from ill patients to those living with or caring for them. According to the Centers for Disease Control and Prevention (CDC), the MERS mortality rate is 30% to 40%.[4] MERS-CoV is mostly confined to the Middle East and currently poses no large threat to those living in the United States.

Bats and other animals remain the primary infection reservoirs for coronaviruses. Most coronaviruses remain nonhuman-based, with just a few affecting humans (**TABLE 1-1**).

When coronaviruses adapt and spread to humans, they can cause illness predominantly in the respiratory system. Patients commonly present with cold- and flu-like symptoms, including fever,

TABLE 1-1 Types of Coronaviruses
Coronaviruses Known to Affect Humans
Human coronavirus (HCoV) 229E
Human coronavirus (HCoV) OC43
Human coronavirus HKU1
Human coronavirus NL63
Middle East respiratory syndrome (MERS)
SARS coronavirus (SARS-CoV, SARS-CoV-2)
Coronaviruses Not Known to Affect Humans
Avian infectious bronchitis virus (IBV)
Bat coronaviruses (eg, SARS-like coronavirus Rp3, HKU2, HKU4, 229-like coronavirus)
Bovine coronavirus (BCoV)
Canine coronavirus (CCoV)
Feline infectious peritonitis virus (FIPV)
Mouse hepatitis virus (MHV)
Porcine epidemic diarrhea virus (PEDV)
Porcine hemagglutinating encephalomyelitis virus (HEV)
Porcine transmissible gastroenteritis virus (TGEV)
Rat coronavirus (RCoV)
Rat sialodacryoadenitis virus (SDAV)
Turkey coronavirus (TCoV)

Data from Greenwood D, Slack R, Barer M: *Medical Microbiology*, ed 18. London: Churchill Livingstone, 2012; and Centers for Disease Control and Prevention: *Human Coronavirus Types*. https://www.cdc.gov/coronavirus/types .html#:~:text=People%20around%20the%20world%20commonly,and%20MERS%2DCoV. Accessed October 6, 2020.

cough, runny nose, and difficulty breathing. Older adults and people with preexisting medical conditions tend to become sicker than their younger, healthier counterparts. In patients with underlying medical conditions such as heart disease, diabetes, hypertension, and immune system compromise, pneumonia may be more likely to develop and some even die from the virus.

How Coronaviruses Spread

Diseases that are transmitted between animals and humans are known as zoonotic. In some cases, coronaviruses can spread from nonhuman hosts to humans, but not from human to human unless the virus adapts. Viruses that do spread from human to human, such as MERS-CoV and SARS-CoV-2, commonly do so through respiratory droplets and aerosolized particles produced during coughing, sneezing, or talking.

It is also possible for people to become infected with coronavirus by touching a fomite, an object or surface contaminated with the virus, and then touching their eyes, nose, or mouth. Fomites can include door handles, tables, countertops, condiment dispensers, pens, and other items in public areas handled by multiple people. Fomite transmission is not considered a primary or even common mode of transmission of COVID-19; however, contact with infectious surfaces still poses a risk of infection.[5]

Although surface contamination is not thought to be the primary mode of transmission, both symptomatic and asymptomatic patients can transmit the virus onto surfaces or to those with whom they come in contact. Once an individual is exposed to the virus, the incubation time—that is, the time it takes for symptoms to develop—can be 2 to 14 days.

COVID-19: A Closer Look

The SARS-CoV-2 virus, which causes COVID-19, is a novel virus, which means it is newly identified. Some of the earliest documented identifications of the virus occurred in December 2019, in the Hubei Province of China. Approximately 24 patients in one community presented with signs and symptoms of lung infection, quickly designated as a novel community-acquired pneumonia (CAP).

The name COVID-19 reveals much about the origin and nature of this disease: *CO* for corona, *VI* for virus, *D* for disease, and *19* for the year it was identified, 2019. The SARS-CoV-2 virus, as with other coronaviruses, was first identified in bats and other animals. When this virus adapted and spread to humans, it transmitted easily to other humans, resulting in a pandemic.

From Disease to Pandemic

With the rapid transmission of SARS-CoV-2, many people became ill in a short time. With communities not knowing exactly what the illness was or how to manage it, hospitals quickly filled up, creating a shortage of hospital beds—specifically, intensive care hospital beds. Medical facilities also experienced a shortage of necessary equipment, such as ventilators. Inadequate supplies of personal protective equipment (PPE) for health care workers meant many were asked to care for patients wearing the same face mask for several days, or until it was visibly soiled. This lack of appropriate PPE put providers at greater risk of becoming ill themselves.

EMS agencies had to evaluate their procedures, both to limit their providers' exposure to the virus and to avoid the risk that providers would become vectors for COVID-19 transmission, spreading the virus as they moved from scene to scene throughout a community. Response protocols in many EMS systems changed dramatically. In March 2020, WHO declared COVID-19 a global pandemic, and countries across the world imposed guidelines to help limit the spread of the illness.

Testing and Diagnosis

COVID-19 is diagnosed by detection of the virus. There are two general methods to obtain a sample for virus detection, and two general methods of conducting the testing. With regard to sampling, one method involves collecting posterior nasal cavity cells with a swab. The swab is gently twisted in the nasopharyngeal cavity for several seconds to collect cells that are then examined for the presence of the virus's RNA. With regard to testing, one method detects the viral antigen directly (antigen testing) and the other (PCR or molecular testing)

Mortality Rates

Initial estimates suggested that the mortality rate of COVID-19 might be as high as 7%, dramatically higher than that of other diseases such as influenza, which has a mortality rate of less than 1% (**TABLE 1-2**). As researchers continue to learn more about COVID-19, and as medical treatment for it has evolved through science and experience, the mortality rate for those infected has become much lower. By September 2020, the CDC calculated the COVID-19 mortality rate at slightly less than 5%. This figure is still in flux, as there is much discussion about the parameters used to calculate the infection and mortality rates.

TABLE 1-2 Flu and COVID-19 Estimates

2019–2020	Influenza (estimated)	COVID-19
Illnesses	39,000,000–56,000,000	7,740,934
Hospitalizations	410,000–740,000	59,728
Deaths	26,000–62,000	214,108

Data from Centers for Disease Control and Prevention: 2019–2020 US Flu Season: Preliminary In-Season Burden Estimates. https://www.cdc.gov/flu/about/burden/preliminary-in-season-estimates.htm. Accessed October 6, 2020. COVIDView Summary for the Week Ending October 3, 2020. https://www.cdc.gov/coronavirus/2019-ncov/covid-data/covidview/index.html. Accessed October 12, 2020; United States COVID-19 Cases and Deaths by State. https://covid.cdc.gov/covid-data-tracker. Accessed October 15, 2020.

The decrease in mortality rate reflects the growing understanding that many people who have COVID-19 have no symptoms or only minor symptoms. Thus, because the total number of people with COVID-19 is higher than the numbers initially reflected, the actual mortality rate is lower. Communities will clarify morbidity and mortality rates as more data become available.

To better understand mortality rates and COVID-19, it is also important to consider excess mortality, a concept that refers to the rate of death during a crisis that is beyond what would be considered normal during that time.

Death rates during a set period can be predicted based on data from previous years. During a pandemic, overall death rates may increase, but the entirety of this increase does not necessarily represent people who died from the pandemic disease itself. In the case of COVID-19, the number of deaths during the pandemic has been higher than would have been expected without the pandemic.

Many of these deaths can be directly attributed to COVID-19, whereas others are only indirectly associated with COVID-19. For example, the stress on the health care system due to COVID-19 may have limited the ability of people with other conditions to receive care. In some instances, people elected not to seek medical care for medical conditions because of concerns about being exposed to COVID-19. In other cases, the economic shutdown imposed to limit spread of the virus resulted in hardship that led to increased suicide rates, decreased ability to afford prescription medications, and other lifestyle changes that resulted in some level of increased mortality. Some deaths from unknown causes in certain communities may have been counted as unrelated to COVID-19 when, in fact, they represented death from pandemic-related viral illness.

For all of these reasons, understanding the true effect of the pandemic on mortality requires a more sophisticated approach than simply measuring COVID-19 confirmed deaths.

uses a technique to amplify the viral load in the sample and then detect the viral genetic material. Antigen testing is generally faster but not as reliable (either positive or negative). PCR testing is much more accurate, but the test must be done in a laboratory and is generally slower. Another method collects cells from a person's saliva instead. A true negative test result suggests that the patient is not currently infected and cannot spread the illness. Some current guidelines allow an individual who tests negative to return to work or school immediately.

Once exposed to an illness, the human body develops antibodies to help prevent illness if exposed to the pathogen again. A blood test can identify the presence of SARS-CoV-2 antibodies, which indicates the patient has been previously exposed to SARS-CoV-2 and may have an immunity to it. This antibody testing provides additional data in determining incidence and prevalence of a disease in a population. However, currently it is not known how long a healthy individual with positive SARS-CoV-2 antibody results would be considered safe from reinfection or what antibody levels are necessary to confer functional immunity from reinfection. Some versions of the test require only a small finger stick to extract blood. The results of the test can be obtained in hours or days, depending on the laboratory or site where the test is conducted.

Although infection and antibody tests are crucial for understanding and controlling the spread of COVID-19, it is essential to recognize the limits of testing. The supply chain of testing products is improving, but some areas still experience delays in both receiving testing supplies and processing the tests. These delays have cascading effects; without test results, workers cannot return to their jobs, students cannot return to school, and contact tracing cannot be conducted to identify people who may have been exposed to individuals who test positive.

In addition, without comprehensive contact tracing, testing provides only a snapshot in time. A negative result today does not mean the person will be negative if tested again tomorrow, if the person has been interacting with others since the time of initial testing or if the person was only recently exposed to the virus at the time of testing.

Also, not all antibody tests are equally useful. In March 2020, the US Food and Drug Administration (FDA) issued a policy allowing developers of serologic tests (antibody tests) to market them once the developer deemed them accurate. Since this policy was introduced, some firms have falsely claimed their tests are FDA-approved and have overstated their accuracy.[6]

It is also important to remember that a COVID-19 test can return false-positive results

(incorrectly indicating that a particular condition or attribute is present) or false-negative results (incorrectly indicating that a particular condition or attribute is absent). A false-positive result can lead to a person being unnecessarily quarantined. Even more concerning, a false-negative result can lead infected patients to believe they can safely interact with others.

Given these variables, it is crucial to interpret COVID-19 test results carefully, following recommendations from the CDC and WHO (**TABLE 1-3**).

Scope of the Disease

When someone becomes infected with SARS-CoV-2, the virus attaches to the same cellular receptors as angiotensin-converting enzyme 2 (ACE-2). Cells with ACE-2 receptors are abundant in the lungs, although these cells also exist throughout the vasculature. Symptoms of COVID-19 may include cough, a loss of smell and/or taste, nausea and vomiting, diarrhea, congestion, sore throat, fatigue, and muscle or body aches.

It is important to note that some patients may not experience classic signs and symptoms, yet are still infected and capable of transmitting the virus to others. A concern with these carriers is the danger of asymptomatic spread. In the absence of symptoms, the infected person may continue to go to work and interact with others in public places, unknowingly exposing others to the virus and further spreading the disease.

Experts are still learning about the damage the SARs-CoV-2 virus is capable of causing. In most cases, as with the common cold caused by a coronavirus, the body's immune system mounts an effective response to the virus and eradicates it, and the patient fully recovers. When healthy people become symptomatic with COVID-19, their symptoms typically last for up to 2 weeks. But even otherwise healthy patients can experience complications, including prolonged symptoms, an extreme overreactive immune response, and even death. In older adults and those with chronic medical conditions such as hypertension and diabetes, these side effects are more common.

Long-term effects of the disease are not yet fully understood and can involve neurologic,

TABLE 1-3 Guidance on Interpreting COVID-19 Test Results

Result	Interpretation	Recommended Action
Viral testing (testing for current infection)		
Positive	*Most likely* you DO currently have an active COVID-19 infection and can give the virus to others.	Stay home and follow CDC guidance on steps to take if you are sick. If you are a health care or critical infrastructure worker, notify your employer of your test result.
Negative	*Most likely* you DO NOT currently have an active COVID-19 infection.	If you have symptoms, you should keep monitoring symptoms and seek medical advice about staying home and if you need to get tested again.
		If you do not have symptoms, you should get tested again only if your medical provider and/or workplace tells you to. *Take steps to protect yourself and others*.
Antibody testing (testing for past infection)		
Positive	You *likely* have HAD a COVID-19 infection.	You may be protected from reinfection (have immunity), but this cannot be said with certainty. Scientists are conducting studies to provide more information. *Take steps to protect yourself and others*.
Negative	You *likely* NEVER HAD (or have not yet developed antibodies to) COVID-19 infection.	You could still get COVID-19. *Take steps to protect yourself and others*.
No test is ever perfect. All tests occasionally result in false-positive results or false-negative results. Results should always be reviewed by a healthcare professional.		

Adapted from Department of Health and Human Services. Guidance on Interpreting COVID-19 Test Results, The White House. https://www.whitehouse.gov/wp-content/uploads/2020/05/Testing-Guidance.pdf. Accessed October 6, 2020.

hematologic, and respiratory sequelae. Some severe cases progress to multiorgan failure or to acute respiratory distress syndrome (ARDS). With ARDS, the lung tissue becomes damaged, the alveoli in the lungs begin to fill with fluid, and the ability to transfer oxygen into the blood is hindered. Patients with ARDS can die secondary to hypoxia. It is possible for patients to die from sepsis because the infection overwhelms their body's defenses (**FIGURE 1-2**).

Most survivors of COVID-19 experience few or no lasting effects. For others, long-term complications can include scarring of the lung tissue (pulmonary fibrosis), which may cause respiratory problems later in life. In some survivors, coagulopathy (abnormal blood clotting), including

disseminated intravascular coagulation (DIC), develops. With DIC, a person's blood clots faster than normal. Clotting factors in the blood are rapidly depleted as a result, eventually leading to an inability to form further clots and then uncontrollable bleeding in some patients. In others, the clotting phase of the illness has been associated with an increased incidence of stroke and myocardial infarction secondary to the COVID-19 illness.

Much more needs to be learned about COVID-19, and research is ongoing. For instance, the disease was initially thought to be nonrelapsing, but a limited study of repeat cases suggests this may not always be true. Some patients in whom COVID-19 was diagnosed and were admitted to hospitals for treatment later experienced a

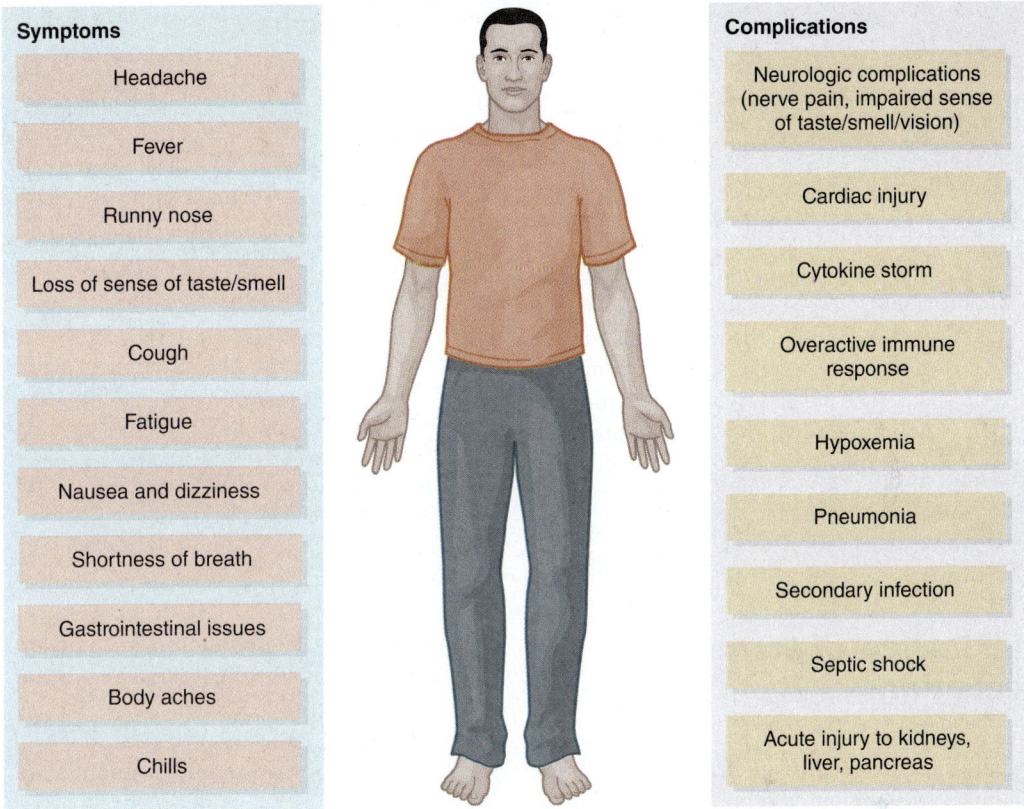

FIGURE 1-2 COVID-19 symptoms and complications.
© Jones & Bartlett Learning.

recurrence of symptoms. During the relapses, the duration of symptoms was slightly shorter and younger, healthier patients required no hospitalization. Older patients with comorbidities required readmission.[7]

The still-evolving body of authoritative knowledge about COVID-19 makes prevention strategies, including both nonpharmacologic interventions (eg, use of face masks and social distancing) and vaccines, crucial in controlling the spread of the virus.

PART 2

Nonpharmacologic Prevention Strategies

The best protection against COVID-19 is to avoid coming in contact with the virus: an almost impossible task if you spend any time in public areas. As an EMS provider, your risk of exposure is heightened as a result of the unique, interactive nature of your work. The virus has demonstrated its capability to spread rapidly and to infect people without producing symptoms; thus, you will sometimes be interacting with patients who do not seem to be infectious. Given the unlikelihood that you will be able to avoid exposure completely, the next best way to prevent contraction is to protect yourself during periods of potential exposure.

Brief Review of Standard Precautions

Staying safe as an EMS provider starts with following approved guidelines for the larger population. Without these commonsense precautions, all people in the community are at risk for contracting contagious illnesses, such as COVID-19.

Keep Your Distance

SARS-CoV-2, like other coronaviruses, is transmitted predominantly through respiratory droplets and aerosolized particles. Because aerosolized particles are smaller and lighter than droplets, they can travel farther and remain suspended in the air for more extended periods. When an infected person sneezes, coughs, talks, or just breathes, droplets and aerosols containing SARS-CoV-2 are dispersed into the air and can travel at least several feet. If these invisible droplets and microdroplets enter another person's eyes, nose, or mouth, that person is now at risk of contracting the illness.

The number of SARS-CoV-2 particles that need to be absorbed or ingested to yield disease is still being researched, but the rapid spread of COVID-19 within communities suggests the number may be relatively low. When SARS-CoV-2 enters the body, the virus begins to replicate within cells. A person's immune system works to stop this replication before it causes significant tissue damage and illness. The ability of a person's body to effectively ward off the virus depends on both the strength of the body's immune system and the viral load, or amount of viral particles in the body. Additional factors, such as the presence of comorbid conditions, play a role. Early in the

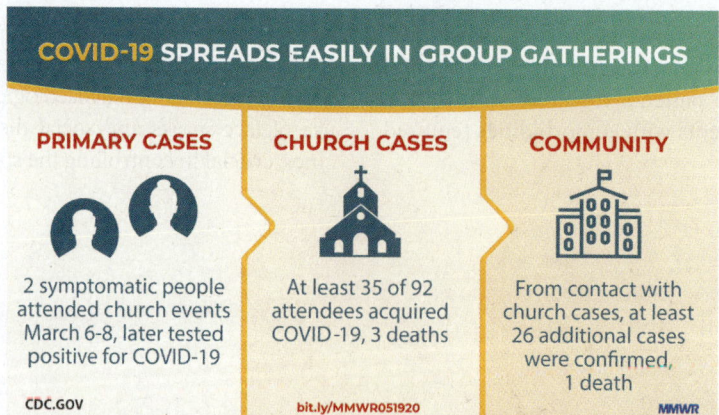

FIGURE 2-1 How one group event impacted multiple COVID-19 transmissions.

Reproduced from James A, Eagle L, Phillips C, et al: High COVID-19 Attack Rate Among Attendees at Events at a Church — Arkansas, March 2020. *MMWR Morb Mortal Wkly Rep 2020*;69:632–635. DOI: http://dx.doi.org/10.15585/mmwr.mm6920e2. Accessed October 15, 2020.

illness, infected people may shed viral particles at a higher rate than later in the illness, after their immune system has been activated.[8] Therefore, all exposures must be taken seriously and evaluated appropriately.

To minimize your exposure, take the following precautions:

- **Keep your physical distance from others.** The greater the distance between an infected person and a noninfected person, the less the chance of exposure. The Centers for Disease Control and Prevention (CDC) recommends maintaining a minimum distance of 6 feet between people in a public space. Keep in mind, the virus can still be spread across that 6-foot space, especially through aerosolized particles. Distance does not prevent transmission of the virus; it just helps to decrease the risk.

- **Avoid group gatherings.** Given the nature of respiratory transmission, it is understandable that when people gather in groups, there is a greater likelihood of virus transmission. Avoiding large groups and gatherings in enclosed places further decreases the possibility of transmission (**FIGURE 2-1**).

Wear a Mask

The CDC recommends wearing a cloth mask when in public. The purpose of cloth masks is primarily source control—that is, to reduce the chance of the wearer spreading respiratory droplets and aerosols. The mask should not inhibit breathing and should cover the nose and mouth completely.

Keep in mind, cloth face masks may not protect the wearer from contracting the illness if exposed. When an infected person wears a cloth face mask, the number of infectious droplets and aerosolized particles released into the surrounding air are reduced.

If a person wearing a cloth mask comes in contact with an infected person not wearing a mask, the infected droplets and particles from the infected person can spread to the mask wearer. Viruses are tiny and can travel through the cloth mask and then be inhaled by the wearer. Additionally, cloth masks rarely make a tight seal around the nose and face, allowing additional routes for transmission. This is why it is important for anyone who goes out in public—especially when physical distancing is not possible—to wear a mask. Masks reduce respiratory droplet transmission between two people most effectively when *both* people are wearing a mask (**FIGURE 2-2**).

Recommendations for properly wearing a cloth mask include the following:

- **Before applying the cloth mask, wash your hands thoroughly for at least 20 seconds.** If the virus was transferred onto your hands, your hands could transfer the virus to your mask, and you may then inhale the virus.

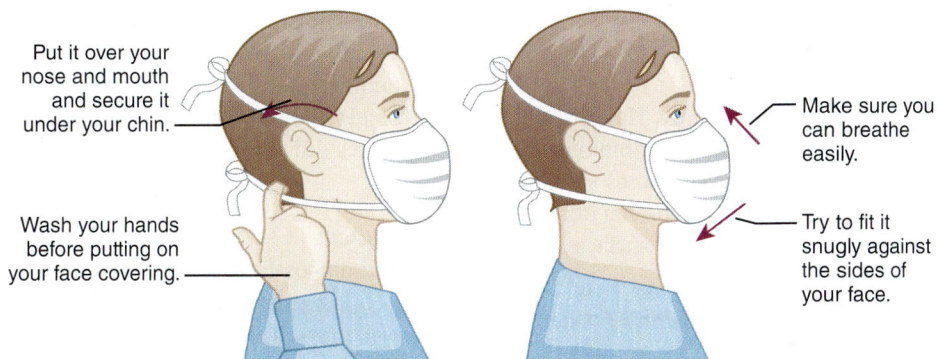

Put it over your nose and mouth and secure it under your chin.

Wash your hands before putting on your face covering.

Make sure you can breathe easily.

Try to fit it snugly against the sides of your face.

FIGURE 2-2 Properly wearing a cloth mask helps prevent disease spread.
© Jones & Bartlett Learning.

- **After washing your hands, place the mask over your nose and under your chin.** The mask should fit as snugly as possible to the side of the face.

- **When removing the mask, do not place it on a potentially contaminated surface.**

- **Wash cloth masks frequently.** Using a washing machine or washing by hand using a mild bleach solution are both effective cleaning methods. Dry the mask by using a clothes dryer or hanging it to air-dry. Be sure to follow manufacturer instructions for cleaning.

Prevent Surface Transmission

It is known that SARS-CoV-2 can live on surfaces, including door handles, tabletops, and writing utensils (such as pens), for long periods. Early evidence suggests the virus can survive up to 24 hours on cardboard, and 2 to 3 days on plastic and stainless steel.[9]

Viruses living on surfaces cannot jump onto people. They travel via a living organism, known as a vector. A vector does not cause disease itself but instead is a conduit for transferring disease from one place to another or one person to another.

People become vectors if they carry the virus and transmit it to a surface through respiratory droplets and aerosolized microdroplets. If an infected person coughs, sneezes, or in any way transfers respiratory emissions to a surface, another person may then touch the surface and acquire the virus. If that person then touches his or her eyes, nose, or mouth, the virus may move to that person's respiratory tract and potentially infect the person.

Precautions to help prevent surface transmissions include the following:

- **Wash your hands frequently.** Hand washing is the most effective method of inhibiting virus transmission from surfaces. Hands should be washed frequently and after coming in contact with potentially contaminated surfaces. Wash your hands as follows:

  1. Place your hands under running water.

  2. Once your hands are wet, use soap to help release the microbes from the skin. There is currently no evidence that using an antiviral soap is more or less effective than regular soap.

  3. Rub your hands together for at least 20 seconds, bringing the soap to a lather. It is essential to scrub your entire hand, including the back of the hand and between the fingers. The area under your fingernails can also harbor bacteria and viruses.

  4. Rinse your hands under clean running water.

  5. Dry your hands with a clean towel, or let your hands air-dry.

- **Avoid touching surfaces unnecessarily.** When in public, such as stores and restaurants, use automatic doors, do not rest or lean on counters, and bring personal pens or styluses instead of using items available to the general public.

- **Wipe and disinfect all commonly touched surfaces.** This process is becoming routine in public spaces. For example, many stores have incorporated the standard of wiping the handles of shopping carts after each use. These habits also should be practiced in private homes and office spaces.

- **Use gloves appropriately.** Some people wear gloves to stop virus transmission when in public. Wearing gloves may limit the transmission of the virus onto the fingers, but the virus will still exist on the glove and can transfer the virus to other objects touched, such as wallets, purses, and eyeglasses. To wear gloves as an effective protective barrier, remove and discard them after touching each potentially contaminated surface, and *before* touching other objects. Keep in mind, inappropriately using gloves can actually help spread the virus.

In addition to following these suggestions, it is important to keep your hands away from your face and mucosal membranes. Avoid rubbing your eyes, licking your fingers, biting your fingernails, and placing your fingers in your nose. Remember, even if hands have been washed thoroughly, the virus may maintain a small presence in the crevices of the hand and under the fingernails. Touching a mucosal membrane may result in a person contracting the virus.

Additional PPE Considerations for EMS Providers

As part of day-to-day activities, health care workers have a higher likelihood of being exposed to people who are knowingly or unknowingly infected with COVID-19. This risk is especially high for workers serving in emergency departments, on ambulances, and in fire departments. For example, a patient experiencing an unrelated emergency (such as a heart attack) may have COVID-19, even if the person is not presenting with COVID-related symptoms.

When providing patient care, you typically cannot maintain a 6-foot distance, and thus have an increased risk of exposure. But you can take extra precautions to avoid becoming infected. Where possible, minimize patient contact until you can assess potential infection or exposure and take appropriate actions, such as masking the patient and/or moving the patient to a well-ventilated area. In all cases, use appropriate protective equipment that is properly cleaned and decontaminated.

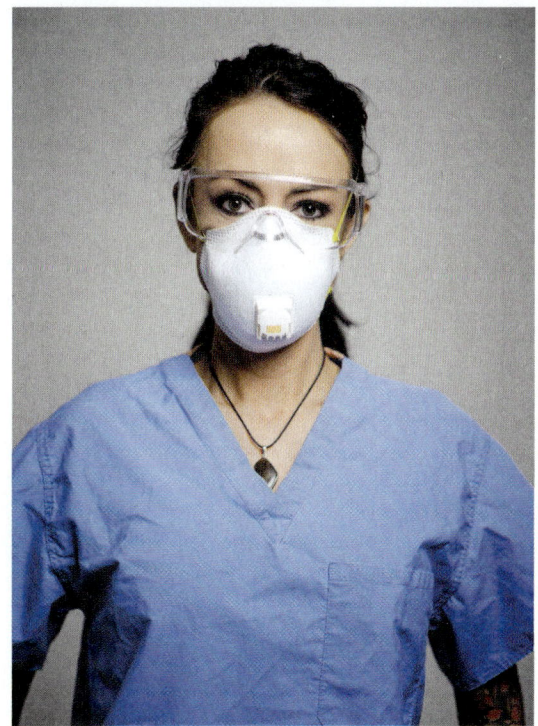

FIGURE 2-3 Wearing a NIOSH-approved mask.
© RichLegg/E+/Getty Images.

Use a NIOSH-Approved Respirator or Face Mask

As mentioned, cloth masks, and even simple surgical masks, do not effectively prevent the wearer from contracting COVID-19. They are useful primarily as a method of source control. For greater protection, the CDC recommends that health care workers who may be exposed to COVID-19 wear a fit-tested N95 filtering respirator or other face piece certified by the National Institute for Occupational Safety and Health (NIOSH) (**FIGURE 2-3**).

The material in an N95 respirator, commonly called an N95 mask, has a tighter weave that more effectively filters out the virus, and the design fits more closely around the nose and mouth. However, its effectiveness requires a correct fit and proper handling:

- **Have your N95 respirator fit-tested.** To effectively block virus droplets from entering your mucous membranes, the respirator should be fitted to your face. Fit-testing is required by law

(OSHA regulation 1910.134) and is commonly done by the provider's employer. It can involve trying several different models to obtain a proper seal. When self-testing a fit, follow recommended guidelines and consider removing any facial hair that interferes with a tight seal. Keep in mind, breathing can be more difficult than usual because of the facial seal and the tight weave of the respirator (**FIGURE 2-4**).

- **Follow facility or agency guidelines regarding N95 respirator disposal or reuse.** Some medical facilities have policies in place to clean and reuse N95 masks and other respirators because of their short supply. If you are asked to reuse an N95 respirator, it should be discarded after it becomes visibly soiled. The CDC does not currently recommend that non–health care workers wear N95 respirators.

If N95 respirators are difficult to obtain due to a supply shortage or other constraints, EMS providers

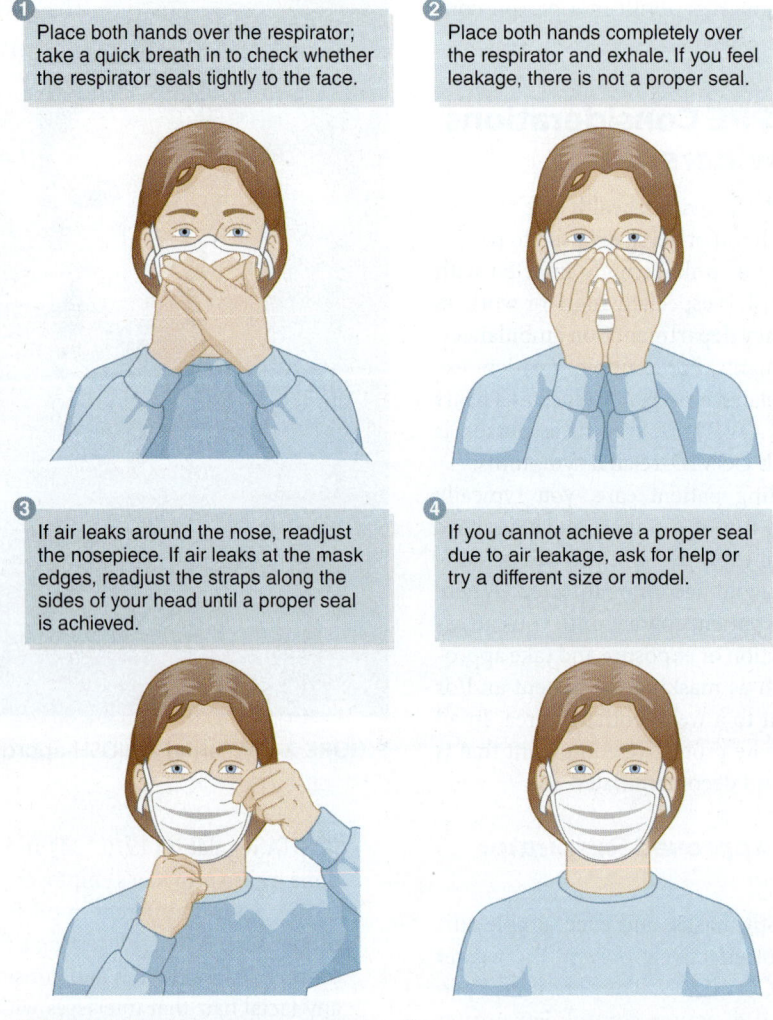

1 Place both hands over the respirator; take a quick breath in to check whether the respirator seals tightly to the face.

2 Place both hands completely over the respirator and exhale. If you feel leakage, there is not a proper seal.

3 If air leaks around the nose, readjust the nosepiece. If air leaks at the mask edges, readjust the straps along the sides of your head until a proper seal is achieved.

4 If you cannot achieve a proper seal due to air leakage, ask for help or try a different size or model.

FIGURE 2-4 Self-testing a respirator fit.
© Jones & Bartlett Learning.

may wear other, equivalent face coverings, such as elastomeric respirators, powered air-purifying respirator (PAPR) devices, or self-contained breathing apparatus (SCBA) face pieces. Elastomeric respirators are half face-covering masks with replaceable filtering cartridges (**FIGURE 2-5**). The masks are commonly made of plastic or rubber and fit the face tightly.

SCBA face pieces are commonly used to enter smoke-filled structures (**FIGURE 2-6**). Although not usually practical, these devices can be used in place of N95 respirators or other face masks when working with patients who are, or may be, positive for COVID-19. Often a filter is attached to the face piece in lieu of the standard air cylinder adapter. Both of these face coverings should be disinfected after every use and in accordance with manufacturer recommendations.

Use Eye Protection, Isolation Gowns, and Gloves

In addition to an N95 respirator, the CDC recommends that health care workers wear eye protection, isolation gowns, and gloves, which need not be sterile (**FIGURE 2-7**).

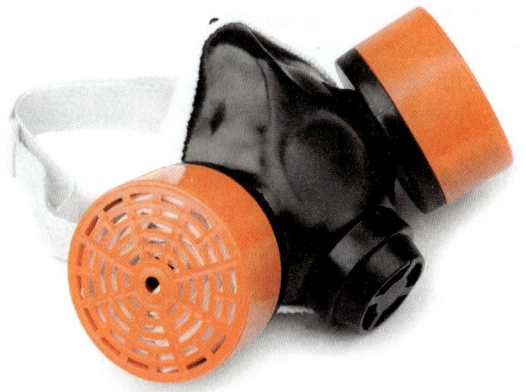

FIGURE 2-5 An elastomeric respirator.
© Anton Starikov/Shutterstock.

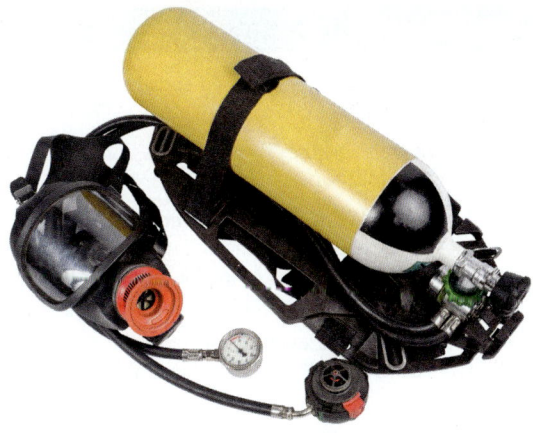

FIGURE 2-6 An SCBA face piece.
© serhii.suravikin/Shutterstock.

Keeping Your Environment Safe

As an EMS provider, you must ensure that you are protecting yourself from COVID-19 and are not exposing others to the virus by unintentionally carrying it on your clothing or equipment.

After caring for a patient, it is vital to clean and disinfect the equipment and ambulance. The PPE worn on a call should be removed and discarded or cleaned between calls. Disposable equipment such as masks, gowns, aprons, and face shields should be replaced.

If you have reusable masks, such as elastomeric respirators, or are asked to reuse your N95 mask, closely adhere to cleaning instructions before wearing them again. If personal clothing becomes contaminated following contact with a patient infected with COVID-19 (or any patient with an infectious disease, for that matter), clean the garments thoroughly as soon as possible. Standard laundering in a washing machine is completely effective for addressing potential contamination due to COVID-19.

Eye protection may consist of goggles or a face shield that covers the front and sides of the face. EMS providers should clean goggles and face shields after each patient interaction, using a recommended disinfectant or alcohol-based wipe.

An isolation gown or apron helps prevent the transmission of the virus to the health care provider's clothing. Before responding to a call, you should know what size gown fits you, and train in donning (putting on) and doffing (removing) the gown. After caring for a patient, the gown or apron should be removed and discarded.

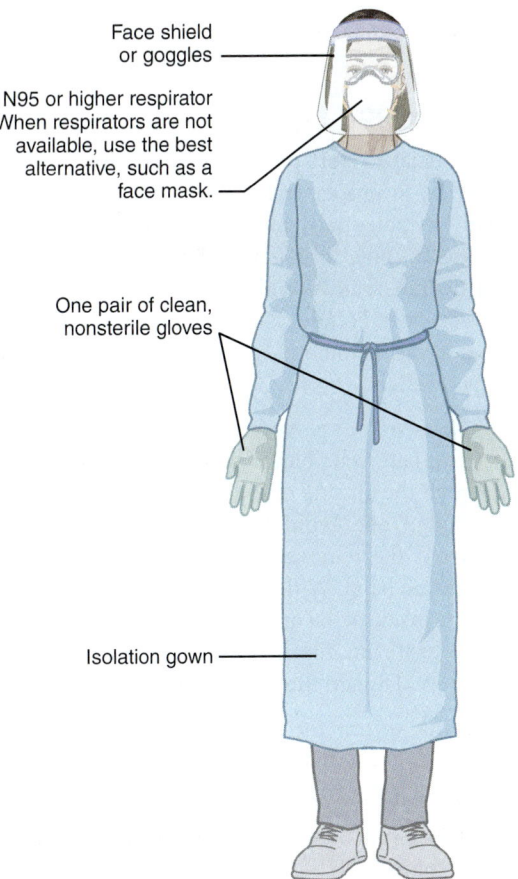

Face shield or goggles

N95 or higher respirator When respirators are not available, use the best alternative, such as a face mask.

One pair of clean, nonsterile gloves

Isolation gown

FIGURE 2-7 Eye protection, isolation gown, and gloves.
© Jones & Bartlett Learning.

PPE Safety

PPE gear is effective *only* when used appropriately. Keep the following in mind:

- Gowns are single-use. They should be discarded after caring for the patient.

- Gowns should not be worn from one patient to another. They should be donned before caring for a patient and doffed after caring for the patient. After removal, the gown should be discarded.

- Gloves should be worn when caring for patients. Like gowns and N95 masks, gloves are single-use and should be discarded after caring for the patient.

- If reusing goggles and face masks, clean them after every use with a recommended disinfectant or alcohol-based wipe.

Remove PPE Equipment Carefully

It is crucial to doff protective gear with caution, adhering to proper technique. After your equipment has potentially touched virus particles, you can easily come in contact with these particles if you do not remove and dispose of items in the correct order. Follow CDC recommendations, and consider using the buddy system to monitor these steps carefully:

1. Remove your gloves first, ensuring not to contaminate your hands. With one gloved hand, grab the outside of the other glove and slowly pull it off. Avoid touching your bare hand. Hold the removed glove in the fist of your gloved hand. With your nongloved hand, grab the inside of the other glove and slowly remove it, capturing the first glove inside the second glove. Discard the gloves in the trash.

2. Untie or tear the gown and remove it downward, from the shoulders first. Discard the gown in the trash.

3. Wash your hands thoroughly for at least 20 seconds.

4. Remove eye protection and face piece. Follow agency or facility policy for disposal, decontamination, or reuse (**FIGURE 2-8**).

Following approved guidelines, both those suggested for the general public and those specific to health care providers, can effectively protect you and those you serve from infection. Visit the CDC and WHO websites for more information and updates on protective equipment and procedures.

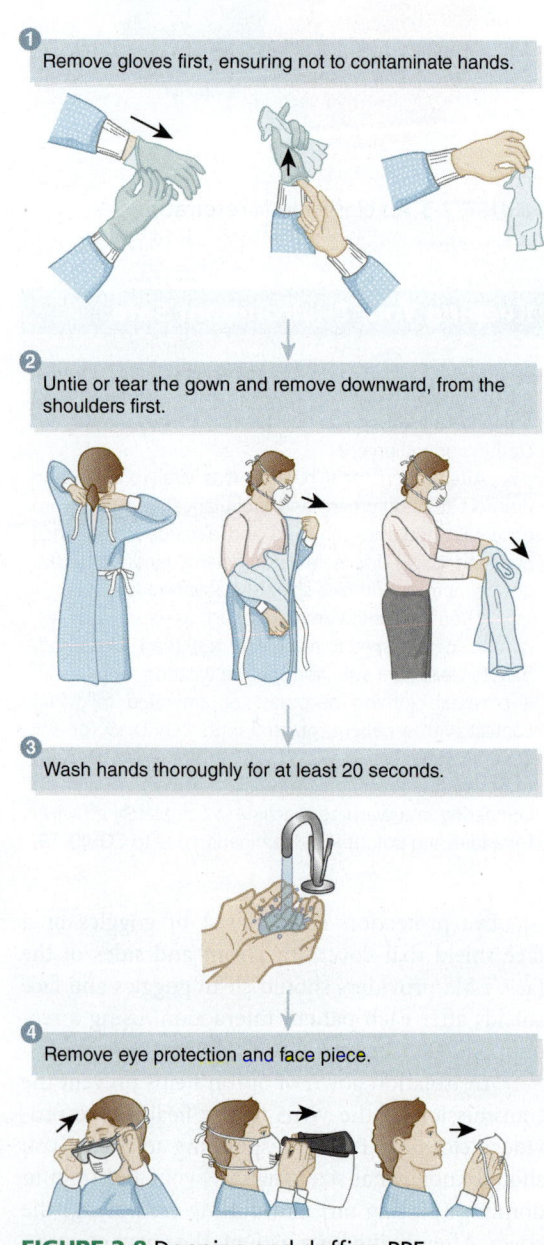

① Remove gloves first, ensuring not to contaminate hands.

② Untie or tear the gown and remove downward, from the shoulders first.

③ Wash hands thoroughly for at least 20 seconds.

④ Remove eye protection and face piece.

FIGURE 2-8 Donning and doffing PPE.
© Jones & Bartlett Learning.

PART 3
Vaccine Development

Since the outbreak of COVID-19, scientists and vaccine specialists have worked to unlock the genetic code of the SARS-CoV-2 virus and develop an effective vaccine. By September 2020, more than 100 vaccine candidates were in development throughout the world, and WHO reported that 40 had advanced to clinical trials.[10]

As an EMS provider, you could be among the first to receive a COVID-19 vaccine and may be tasked with administering the vaccine to the community (**FIGURE 3-1**). Reviewing the course of vaccine development, and understanding the range of candidates being tested, will help prepare you to implement your agency's policies and make sound decisions about your own health.

Typical Course of Development

Developing a COVID-19 vaccine involves the same basic steps used when developing other vaccines:

- Exploratory stage
- Preclinical stage
- Clinical development
- Regulatory review and approval
- Manufacturing
- Quality control

As a solution to the global pandemic, steps are being taken to expedite the COVID-19 vaccine process (**FIGURE 3-2**). In the United States, this expedited process requires condensing and overlapping some phases while maintaining strict review and quality control by the FDA.

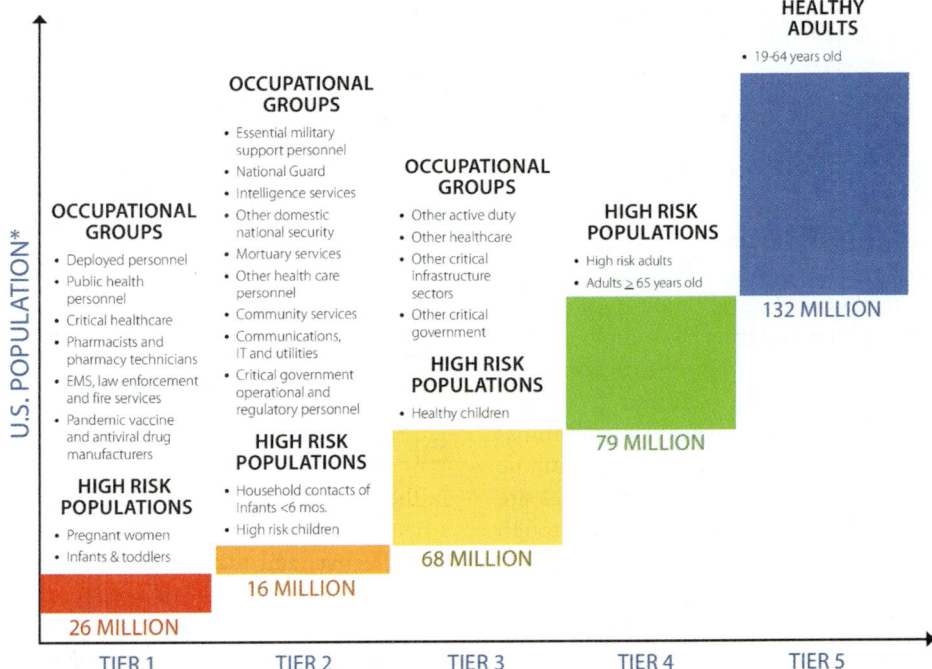

FIGURE 3-1 Tiered vaccine administration structure for high or very high pandemic severity.

* Based on 2015 US population of 321 million people.

Reproduced from Centers for Disease Control and Prevention. Allocating and Targeting Pandemic Influenza Vaccine During an Influenza Pandemic. U.S. Department of Health and Human Services. https://www.cdc.gov/flu/pandemic-resources/pdf/2018-Influenza-Guidance.pdf. 2018. Accessed October 8, 2020.

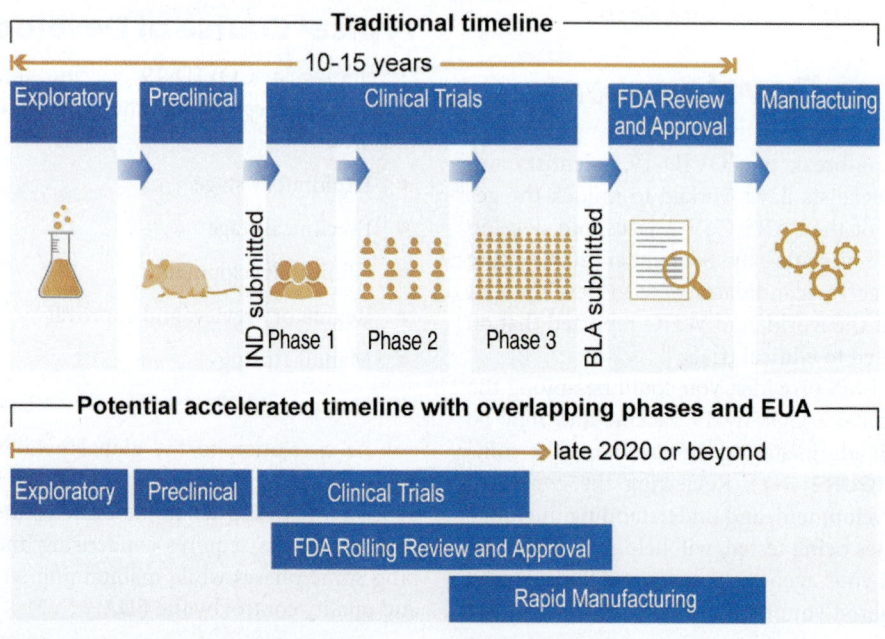

FIGURE 3-2 Timelines for vaccine development.

Abbreviations: BLA, Biologics License application; EUA, Emergency Use Authorization; FDA, Food and Drug Administration; IND, Investigational New Drug.

Government Accountability Office (GAO). Science & Tech Spotlight: COVID-19 Vaccine Development - GAO-20-583SP. May 26, 2020.

Exploratory and Preclinical Stages

These initial stages involve lab research and animal studies. If a virus is known to scientists, the objective after genome sequencing is to determine how to get the human body to build immunity to the disease without suffering its symptoms. For example, with a typical intranasal flu vaccine, an attenuated virus—one that has been genetically altered so it cannot cause disease—is administered. Once exposed, the body elicits an immune response in the local tissue, and antibodies are built against the virus that circulate through the body.

Other vaccines take a surface protein, a specific protein found on the virus and unique to the virus, and expose the immune system so antibodies develop against that protein. Because that protein is located only on the virus that causes the disease, the body builds immunity and destroys that protein if the immune system recognizes it, thus eliminating the virus.

If the virus is unknown to scientists, this exploratory process can be much more tedious, as the virus has to be safely replicated and analyzed prior to determining which type of vaccine may be most effective. Typically this process can last 3 to 6 years. Once a vaccine has been developed in the lab and safely tested on animals, it reaches clinical development and is ready for human testing.

Clinical Development

In the United States, all vaccines must go through a rigorous approval process to ensure they are safe and effective, and that the benefits outweigh the risks. Typically, this stage of development involves three phases (**FIGURE 3-3**).

Before official testing can begin, the FDA, which oversees vaccine testing, requires the vaccine to be inspected and licensed by its review committee. Following this initial review, phase 1 requires a vaccine to be administered to approximately 20 to 100 volunteers. Starting with a small group enables

How a New Vaccine Is Developed, Approved, and Manufactured

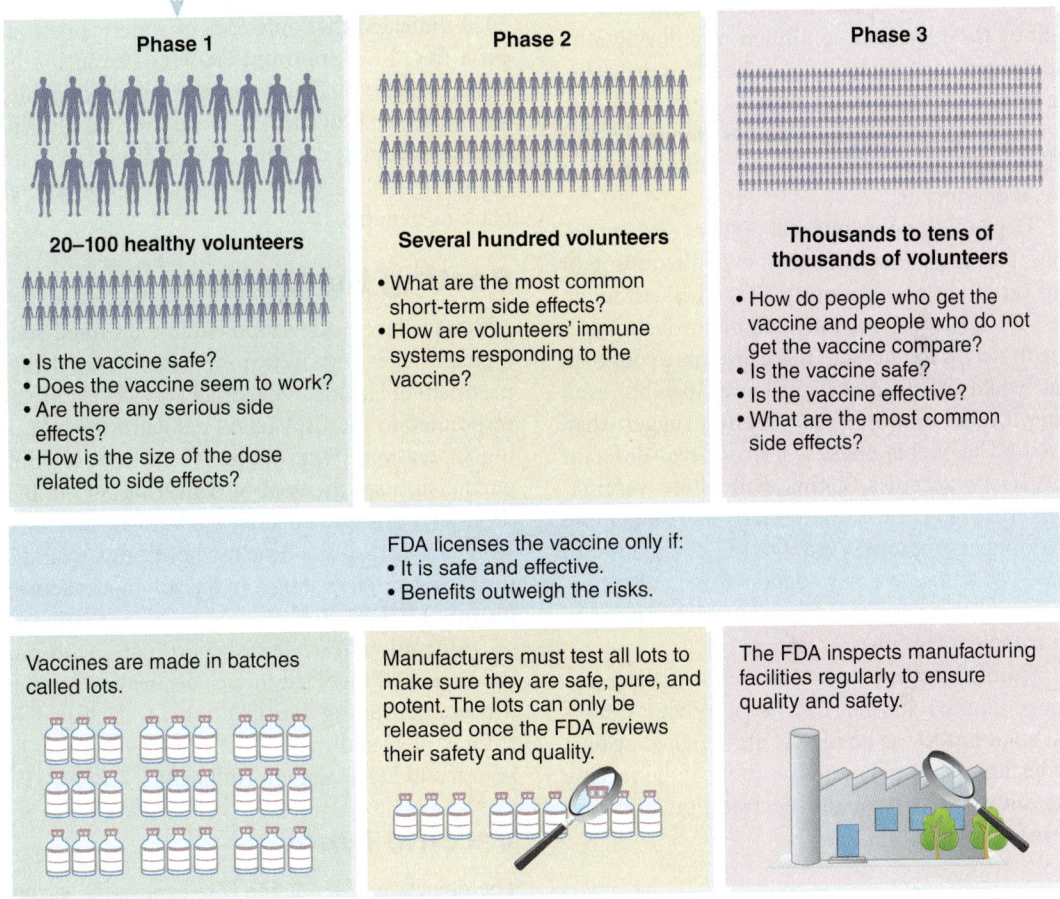

The Food and Drug Administration (FDA) sets rules for the three phases of clinical trials to ensure the safety of the volunteers. Researchers test vaccines with adults first.

Phase 1

20–100 healthy volunteers

- Is the vaccine safe?
- Does the vaccine seem to work?
- Are there any serious side effects?
- How is the size of the dose related to side effects?

Phase 2

Several hundred volunteers

- What are the most common short-term side effects?
- How are volunteers' immune systems responding to the vaccine?

Phase 3

Thousands to tens of thousands of volunteers

- How do people who get the vaccine and people who do not get the vaccine compare?
- Is the vaccine safe?
- Is the vaccine effective?
- What are the most common side effects?

FDA licenses the vaccine only if:
- It is safe and effective.
- Benefits outweigh the risks.

Vaccines are made in batches called lots.

Manufacturers must test all lots to make sure they are safe, pure, and potent. The lots can only be released once the FDA reviews their safety and quality.

The FDA inspects manufacturing facilities regularly to ensure quality and safety.

FIGURE 3-3 Typical testing process for a new vaccine.
Modified from Centers for Disease Control and Prevention. 2018. Provider Resources for Vaccine Conversations With Parents: Ensuring the Safety of Vaccines in the United States. https://www.cdc.gov/vaccines/hcp/conversations/ensuring-safe-vaccines.html. Accessed October 8, 2020.

researchers to determine human response and side effects in a more controlled manner.[11]

If a vaccine meets the safety criteria of phase 1, it moves on to phase 2, where it is given to several hundred volunteers. The vaccine is then evaluated for short-term side effects and immune system response.[11] Typically, phases 1 and 2 take at least 3 months but may last years, as those who received the vaccine are monitored to compare them with patients who did not receive the vaccine or with those who received a placebo instead of the vaccine.

In phase 3, the pool of recipients widens yet again, typically to tens of thousands of people. The participants are monitored to determine the vaccine's effectiveness and side effects and to compare the vaccine recipients with a control group who received a placebo.[11] This final phase can take several months to several years.

Review and Approval

Following successful completion of the trial phases by a vaccine's development groups, each country can elect to approve it for human use. In the United States, review and approval involve rigorous oversight by the FDA and continued monitoring after widespread use. You likely have heard of drugs being recalled or taken off the market because of consequences not fully explored in the testing phase or only recognized after years of use. Although this is rare, it does occur.

Depending on its internal policies and regulations, a country may choose to expedite testing or skip certain phases of testing altogether. Although the COVID-19 vaccine may well be the fastest vaccine to the hit the market, there are some countries that would like to make vaccine availability even faster. In fact, multiple news reports suggest that, based on favorable phase 2 trials of two different COVID-19 vaccines, China will allow vaccinations to be given to some military personnel and government employees prior to the completion of phase 3.[12] Other reports suggest Russia also may provide a China-based vaccine to citizens prior to the completion of phase 3 testing.

Conflicting reports on vaccine use in these and other countries continue to emerge. What is clear is that solutions to the pandemic are weighed against the health of the public and the safety of the vaccine and can vary based on culture, tradition, and government policy.[13]

Manufacturing and Quality Control

After the review process is complete and government agencies approve the new vaccine, it can be manufactured and distributed to licensed facilities. This may sound like a quick part of the process, but manufacturing a sufficient quantity of the medium, syringes, needles, and packaging—all under safety control—takes time. Pharmaceutical companies typically have years to prepare the supply chain for a new vaccine, yet the timelines proposed for the COVID-19 vaccine require mere months.

After preparation and shipment, which will likely occur in batches, the public must be vaccinated. Although most of the population will obtain the vaccine from their health care provider, some citizens will require more convincing. As a health care provider, you may be looking forward to getting vaccinated, but a poll conducted in July 2020 indicated that only 65% of Americans would get a free, FDA-approved COVID-19 vaccine if it were available.[14] Thus, a public health campaign, similar to what occurs every year for the flu shot, will be essential, wherein health care officials and public figures advocate for immunization and explain its benefits.

Beating the Clock

Although vaccine development in the United States typically takes anywhere from 5 to 20 years, the Department of Health and Human Services (HHS) has responded to the COVID-19 pandemic by launching Operation Warp Speed.[15] This private-public partnership set the goal of delivering 300 million doses of a safe and effective COVID-19 vaccine by January 2021. If this timeline holds, this would be the fastest progression from disease to a vaccine in history (**FIGURE 3-4**).

Operation Warp Speed coordinates with multiple agencies involved in the vaccine development process, including the CDC, FDA, National Institutes of Health, and Biomedical Advanced Research and Development Authority.[15]

Vaccine Types

The objective of a vaccine is to expose the vaccine recipient's immune system to the virus or a portion of the virus in order to trigger a response without causing the illness. Several different types of vaccines are currently under development by manufacturers throughout the world. Although it may seem counterintuitive for multiple candidates to simultaneously enter the testing phase, this practice is common and presents multiple approaches (**TABLE 3-1**).

The most likely candidates include vaccinations that introduce an altered form of the virus, introduce a surface protein found on the virus, or introduce instructions for making a protein found on the virus.

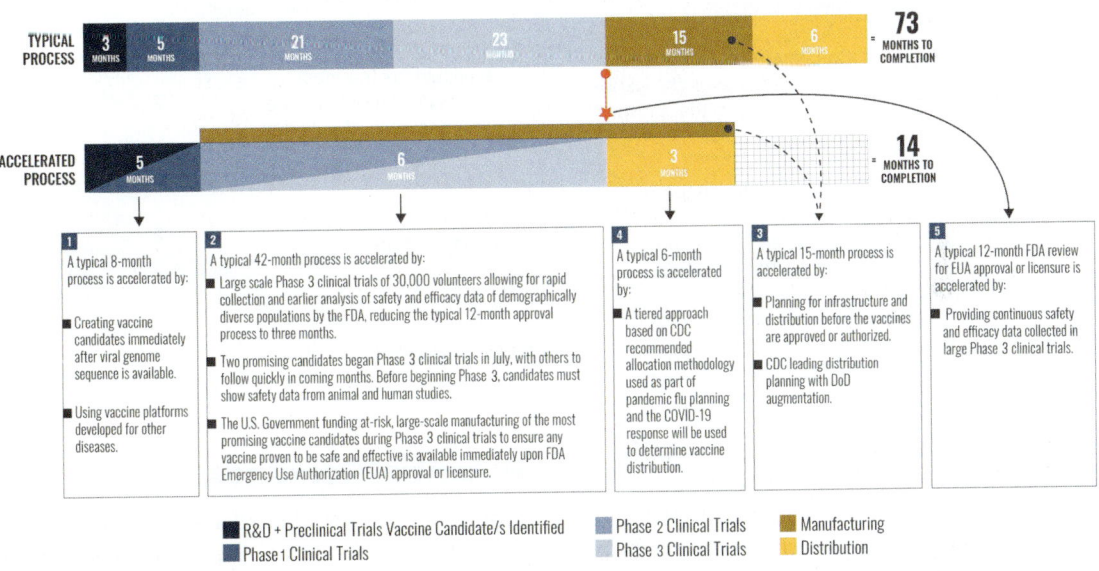

FIGURE 3-4 Accelerated vaccine process for Operation Warp Speed.

Abbreviations: CDC, Centers for Disease Control and Prevention; DoD, Department of Defense; FDA, Food and Drug Administration; R&D, Research and development
Reproduced from US Department of Defense. 2020. Operation Warp Speed: Accelerated Vaccine Process. https://www.defense.gov/Explore/Spotlight/Coronavirus/Operation-Warp-Speed/. Accessed October 8, 2020.

Viral- and vector-based vaccines introduce a version of the SARS-CoV-2 virus, modified to be either dead or unable to replicate, to the recipient. For example, the conventional flu vaccine delivers an inactivated virus. One type of viral COVID-19 vaccine uses the adenovirus as the virus vector. This virus otherwise causes the common cold in humans; however, when used as a vaccine vector, it does not cause illness. In fact, the adenovirus is modified to produce only a protein specific to the coronavirus, produced in a few human cells, and thus elicit a localized immune response in the recipient.[16]

Messenger RNA (mRNA) vaccines skip the step of having the SARS-CoV-2 virus invade a human cell's DNA. Instead, an mRNA vaccine sends instructions to the cells, encoding a message to make proteins specific to the coronavirus. Once the mRNA is taken up by a small number of the vaccine recipient's cells, the protein is produced and the immune response targets the foreign protein. After targeting the protein, the immune system builds memory and defends the body against any virus cells that have the same surface protein.[17]

Another notable virus-based vaccine is a recombinant vesicular stomatitis virus-vectored vaccine. It uses a virus with replication abilities to deliver antigen-producing genes from the coronavirus into human cells. The virus vector incorporates genes from the coronavirus that can be replicated in the recipient. In essence, this process

TABLE 3-1 Representative Approaches to a COVID-19 Vaccine			
Approach	**Description**	**Candidate Types Include**	**Number of Proposed Doses**
Nonreplicating viral vector	Utilizing another virus to introduce COVID-19 virus proteins into the host to elicit an immune response and build immunity.	• Recombinant vesicular stomatitis virus-vectored • Adenovirus	1–2
Inactivated	Coronavirus is introduced into the host; however, the genes are modified so that the virus cannot replicate.	• Limited information available, as the most promising candidates are being developed outside of the US	2
RNA	Instructions to generate corona-virus surface proteins are introduced into the host to elicit an immune response.	• mRNA • Protein subunits	2

Abbreviations: mRNA, messenger RNA; RNA, ribonucleic acid
Data from World Health Organization Draft Landscape of COVID-19 Candidate Vaccines. https://www.who.int/publications/m/item/draft-landscape-of-covid-19-candidate-vaccines. Accessed October 9, 2020.

creates a small amount of the virus, but with only the genes needed to recognize the coronavirus, not those that allow it to replicate. By using a virus with replication capability, in which the recipient's immune system will respond, a more sustained immunogenic response may be produced, limiting the number of required vaccinations. This type of vaccine has also been used to develop a vaccine to the Zaire ebolavirus.[17]

Potential Readiness

Promising vaccine candidates are progressing through clinical testing, but questions remain about whether a vaccine will be readily available by the beginning of 2021. Issues such as efficacy, side effects, adverse reactions, number of doses, availability to the general public, and length of immunity must all be weighed.

PART 4
Treatment Strategies

As of October 2020, definitive treatments for COVID-19 are in development. Clinical trials of antivirals, channel blockers, and other approaches are under way, and outcome evidence from the studies is being analyzed and peer-reviewed. Some promising studies include the following:

- **SIMPLE, CARAVAN, and ACTT-1, -2, and -3.** Based in the United States, these multicenter randomized controlled trials (RCTs) are studying remdesivir in different settings.

- **RECOVERY.** This study, based in the United Kingdom (Oxford), is exploring use of dexamethasone/azithromycin/tocilizumab/convalescent plasma.

- **REMAP-CAP.** This international collaborative effort is studying multiple treatments for all community-acquired pneumonia.

- **CATALYST.** Based in the United Kingdom (Birmingham), this study is investigating multiple medications to decrease intensive care unit (ICU) admissions.

- **REALIST.** This study, based in Ireland (Belfast), is investigating umbilical stem cell therapy.

- **I-SPY.** Based in Japan, this study is examining several repurposed medications, including a bradykinin antagonist.

- **DART.** This study, based in the United States (Johns Hopkins University), is investigating the effectiveness of decitabine.

- **ACTIV series.** Based in the United States, these multicenter RCTs are studying heparin and anticoagulation therapies.

Jumping to premature conclusions about these treatments can ultimately result in delays and even poor outcomes. Many pharmaceutical treatments in the trial phase have significant side effects to patients. Properly addressing all issues and developing widely effective treatments can take months or years, even on a fast-track schedule.

For EMS providers, it is important to align with approved treatment protocols while understanding limitations in the medical community. Current treatment plans for people with mild symptoms of COVID-19 include self-isolation at home, rest, and fluid intake. Treatments for those with severe symptoms requiring hospitalization focus on supporting ventilation and circulation by providing fluids and oxygen.

EMS protocols often involve specific devices and PPE considerations when managing a patient's oxygenation and fluid level requirements. Critical COVID-19 patients may need aggressive hemodynamic and ventilatory support, including invasive airways, positive pressure ventilation (PPV) devices, and pharmacologic blood pressure support. For nonintubated patients, limited studies suggest that placing the patient in a prone position (proning) can help improve respiratory and final outcomes, though more research is needed.[18] There is no evidence as of yet of any benefit in placing patients in a prone position for short periods of time, such as the time periods associated with typical EMS transports. The risks of limiting access to the patient's airway and limiting the ability to monitor the patient may outweigh the benefit of prone positioning in most EMS scenarios.

Diagnosis

Pneumonia is a dangerous lung infection that can, as in the case of COVID-19, be deadly. Those at highest risk are very young children and older adults. Pneumonias are classified as viral, bacterial, or fungal. Viral and bacterial pneumonias are more common than fungal and can spread from person to person through the inhalation of droplets and aerosols. All three types can also exist concurrently.

A systematic review in 2020 of patient care records revealed that between 10% and 29% of traditional pneumonia patients will have both bacterial and viral infections simultaneously.[19] A 2016 systematic review and meta-analysis of 31 published pneumonia studies included more than 10,000 patients and drew similar conclusions, showing that approximately 25% of patients had both viral and bacterial infections.[20] Despite this trend, early cases of this

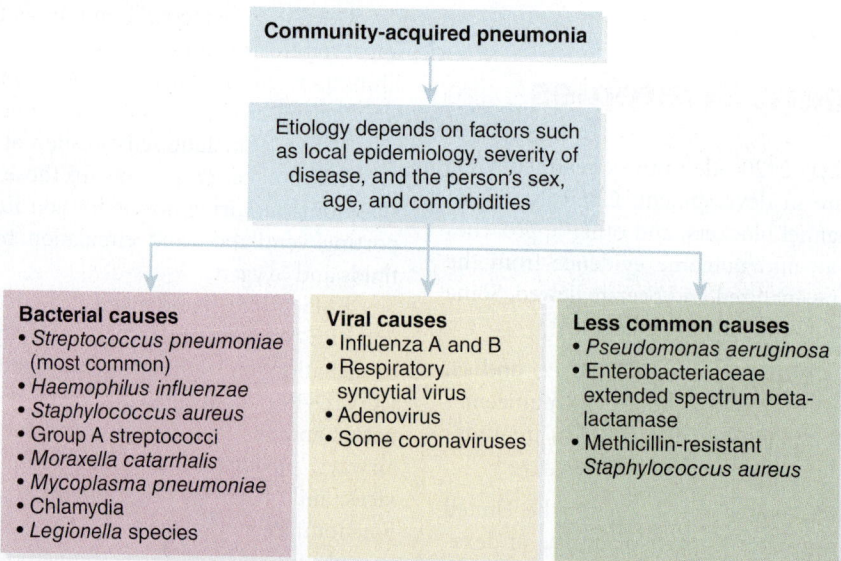

FIGURE 4-1 Distinguishing among community-acquired pneumonias.

Used with permission from Carl Heneghan, Oxford COVID-19 Evidence Service Team, Centre for Evidence-Based Medicine, Nuffield Department of Primary Care Health Sciences, University of Oxford, 2020.

novel CAP (COVID-19) did *not* frequently demonstrate coexisting bacterial pneumonia. Distinguishing the origin was crucial in providing the right care to each patient at the right time (**FIGURE 4-1**).

The most common origins of pneumonia often can be ruled in or out based on clinical presentation and diagnostic testing. Rapid flu swabs are usually performed first and return results within 5 to 15 minutes. Several different microbes can cause bacterial pneumonia, which can be cultured through sputum samples. Sputum tests take longer to provide results but are still extremely important.

Bacterial pneumonias are one of the most common triggers for sepsis, which can progress quickly to septic shock. The Surviving Sepsis Campaign, from the Society of Critical Care, describes a bundle of care called early goal-directed therapy for these patients. This bundle includes early fluid, early antibiotics, and vasopressors when indicated.

When differentiating between viral and bacterial pneumonias, it is helpful to compare and contrast clinical symptoms and diagnostic tests (**TABLE 4-1**). Disease progression rates often differ between COVID-19 patients and patients with more traditional bacterial pneumonia. The presence of discolored or foul-smelling sputum is more often seen in bacterial pneumonia. Though fever can be present in both, it more often results from bacterial pneumonia.

Treatment: An Evolving Set of Strategies

Initially, sepsis was of central concern for patients critically ill with COVID-19 because of high mortality and the association with pneumonia. However, respiratory failure and multiple organ failure often occurred in the absence of bacterial pneumonia. Today, the central concerns in treating COVID-19 patients include respiratory failure, so-called cytokine storm, and certain types of coagulopathy, including disseminated intravascular coagulation.

Respiratory Failure

The most common inflammatory markers of COVID-19 are tachycardia and tachypnea. In the early months of the COVID-19 pandemic, early respiratory failure and ARDS appeared to develop in patients. Radiographic studies of COVID-19 patients often revealed bilateral opacities (**FIGURE 4-2**).

TABLE 4-1 Differentiating COVID-19 From Bacterial Pneumonia	
COVID-19/Viral Pneumonia More Commonly:	**Bacterial Pneumonia More Commonly:**
Presents with a history of typical COVID-19 symptoms for about a week (slow/insidious onset)	Becomes rapidly unwell after only a few days (acute onset)
Has severe muscle pain (myalgia) Experiences loss of sense of smell (anosmia) or taste	Does not have a history of typical COVID-19 symptoms
Causes shortness of breath but has no pleuritic pain	Has pleuritic pain
Causes bilateral positive lung findings	Causes unilateral positive lung findings
Causes typically lower temperature and tachycardia or tachypnea out of proportion to the temperature	Causes typically higher temperature
Causes a paucity of physical findings on pulmonary exam disproportionate to the level of disability (ie, patient appears sicker than their lungs sound)	Has purulent sputum
Has a history of exposure or known suspected COVID-19 through home, workplace, or community spread	Has comorbid bacterial infections

Used with permission from Carl Heneghan, Oxford COVID-19 Evidence Service Team, Centre for Evidence-Based Medicine, Nuffield Department of Primary Care Health Sciences, University of Oxford, 2020.

Computed tomography (CT) scans with bilateral ground-glass opacities became a hallmark of this disease. This radiographic pattern is a marker for fluid filling the lungs. When fluid invades the alveoli, exchange of oxygen and carbon dioxide is inhibited.

Figure 4-2 shows the following:

- **Scan A.** 56-year-old woman with moderate COVID-19. CT image shows pulmonary fibrosis in both lungs (see white boxes).

- **Scan B.** 37-year-old man with moderate COVID-19. CT image shows mixed ground glass opacity (see white box).

- **Scan C.** 32-year-old woman with moderate COVID-19. CT image shows thickening with pleural adhesion (see white arrow).

- **Scan D.** 50-year-old woman with severe COVID-19. CT image shows ground glass opacities in both lungs (see white boxes).

- **Scan E.** 59-year-old woman with severe COVID-19. CT image shows ground glass opacities (see white box) and consolidation

with air bronchogram in the right lung (see black arrow).

- **Scan F.** 65-year-old man with severe COVID-19. CT image shows bronchial wall thickening, and abnormal widening of the airways (see black arrow). Vascular enlargement is also apparent (see white arrows). The white boxes also show pulmonary tissue thickening in both lungs.

Initial respiratory management targets maintaining an adequate level of oxygen saturation (92% to 96%). Many early COVID-19 observational reports and studies identified patients who presented with hypoxia disproportionate to their dyspnea. Subsequently, the phrase "happy hypoxia" started to appear in the differential diagnosis for COVID-19. This paradoxical concept is not new. It first appeared in pulmonary/ARDS literature to describe patients who did not appear short of breath but whose oxygen saturation levels measured low (or extremely low). High-flow nasal cannulas and noninvasive positive pressure ventilation have become first-line treatments for these symptoms.

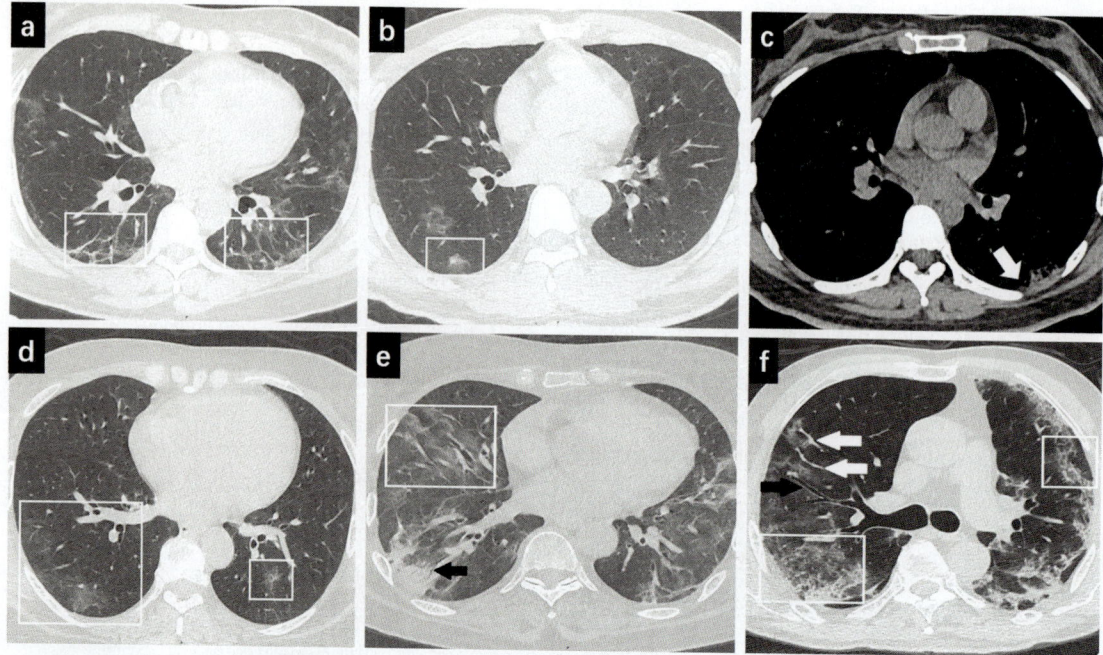

FIGURE 4-2 Ground-glass opacities in COVID-19 patient scans.

Reproduced from Fu Z, Tang N, Chen Y, et al. CT features of COVID-19 patients with two consecutive negative RT-PCR tests after treatment. *Sci Rep* 2020;10:11548. https://covid19.elsevierpure.com/en/publications/ct-features-of-covid-19-patients-with-two-consecutive-negative-rt

High-flow nasal cannulas are not just regular cannulas turned up high. These specialized nasal cannula systems, using devices such as the Fisher & Paykel Optiflow or Vapotherm Precision Flow, can deliver 50 to 60 liters per minute of warm, humidified oxygen (**FIGURE 4-3**).

The warmth and humidity help decrease the inflammation that can occur because of traditional nasal cannula or nonrebreathing systems that are both cold and dry. This type of device also helps maintain the ciliary function in the cells that line the respiratory tract. This type of respiratory assistance does not heal or cure COVID-19; rather, it supports the body long enough to hopefully allow it to recover.

As the respiratory symptoms increase in severity, the treatments and interventions also become increasingly aggressive. Proning is one bridging strategy that can help prevent the need for invasive ventilation. When the alveoli begin to collapse or fill with fluid, the patient may feel increasingly

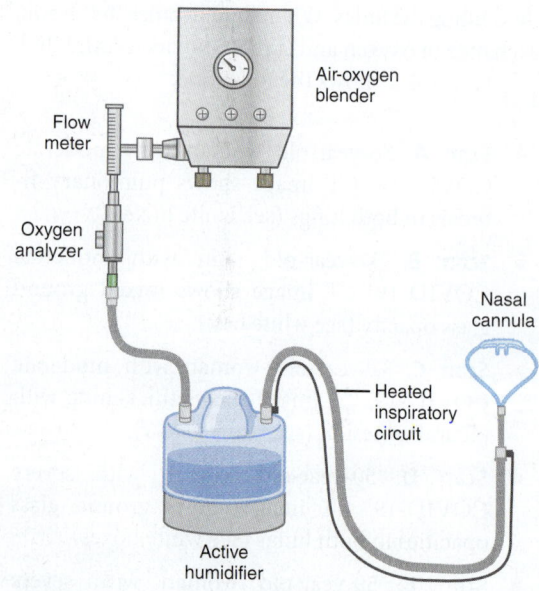

FIGURE 4-3 A high-flow nasal cannula.

© Jones & Bartlett Learning.

short of breath. By positioning the patient in the prone position, the posterior rib cage can expand with greater volume. Several observational studies performed in Italy have shown that proning can increase alveolar recruitment and improve oxygenation and ventilation. This treatment has been evolving for several years in the ICU as one solution to patients with refractory ARDS. In the studies, the patient usually was intubated, and large equipment was required for the procedure every few hours. In the COVID-19 patient, proning is sometimes helpful when the patient is still conscious and able to self-prone. However, the experiences of some clinicians suggest that proning can improve outcomes for severe COVID-19 patients regardless of the oxygen delivery method, invasive or noninvasive.[21]

Proning can be combined with noninvasive ventilation. Continuous positive airway pressure (CPAP) has been a point of uncertainty in COVID-19 protocols since the beginning of the outbreak. Initially, many medical directors and administrators were advising departments to limit the use of CPAP due to the aerosolizing nature of the device. As the disease pathology becomes better understood, and the filter devices become more widely available, CPAP has seen a return to many treatment protocols. CPAP can be combined with

proning to help prevent further respiratory decline and the need for invasive ventilation.

Patients in whom ARDS or respiratory failure develops will often require invasive ventilation by endotracheal intubation. These patients require increasing positive end-expiratory pressure (PEEP) to keep the alveoli open and to maintain adequate oxygenation. According to an early 2020 study, ARDS "is the most common indication for transferring patients with COVID-19 to the ICU and the major cause of death in this patient population."[22] The study also found that any clinical improvement usually occurs after week 2.

Up to this point, because pneumonia in the ICU had been primarily bacterial in nature, many critical care physicians and staff used guidance from the studies generated from the Society of Critical Care Medicine and the Surviving Sepsis Campaign. These two organizations created a joint recommendation for COVID-19 ICU admissions and treatment pathways (**TABLE 4-2**).

Cytokine Storm

One of the contributors to ARDS development is the downstream effect of the inflammatory pathway. Interstitial and pulmonary tissues are damaged from a massive release of cytokines, which are small signal proteins that are released

TABLE 4-2 Recommendations for Managing COVID-19 With Hypoxia		
Severity	**Action**	**Consider**
Acute/failure	• Endotracheal intubation • Practice infection control • Minimize staff	• Video-laryngoscope • Most experienced airway provider
Moderate/subacute	• Monitor closely for worsening • Target SpO$_2$ 92%–96% • Take infection control precautions	• Humidified oxygen • High-flow nasal cannula • NIPPV/CPAP
DO NOT DELAY INTUBATION IF CONDITION DECLINES		

Abbreviations: CPAP, continuous positive airway pressure; NIPPV, Noninvasive positive pressure ventilation; SpO$_2$, oxygen saturation

Based on resources from the Society of Critical Care Medicine and Surviving Sepsis Campaign.

by cells during the inflammatory and immune cascade.

These cellular cascades operate much like the valves in an air/oxygen tank-filling cascade. When the SARS-CoV-2 invades, it takes over the signaling system and essentially opens all the valves at once, flooding the surrounding tissue with the cytokines. This process is referred to as a cytokine storm. In a patient with COVID-19, "the inflammatory cytokine storm is closely related to the development and progression of ARDS."[23] Historically, ARDS is an extremely critical state that is often associated with poor patient outcomes. In COVID-19 patients, researchers found "the serum levels of cytokines to be significantly increased in patients with ARDS," with the degree of increase being "positively correlated with mortality rate."[23]

Early case reviews suggested that the bigger the cytokine storm, the higher the mortality rate. Larger studies are starting to show a less dramatic cytokine response in patients with COVID-19 versus patients with ARDS.[24] This finding has resulted in a downshift in some treatments targeting the cytokine cascade. However, there are still some significant overlaps in the presentation and treatments for these two pathologies, so the concept of cytokine storm in COVID-19 has not yet been entirely abandoned.

Related Coagulopathies

In addition to the pathologies discussed thus far, at least two pathologic coagulation processes appear to occur in critically ill COVID-19 patients. As one study found, "In the microcirculation of the lung and potentially other organs, there is local direct vascular and endothelial injury-producing microvascular clot formation."[25] In the systemic circulation, there is hypercoagulability and hyperactivation of fibrinogen, creating the potential for thrombosis and significant downstream effects, such as pulmonary embolism, stroke, or heart attack. A high index of suspicion for COVID-19 should be maintained in all patients presenting with conditions involving clot formation or embolization.

Although disseminated intravascular coagulation is a hallmark of late sepsis, COVID-19 coagulopathy is markedly different. Providers draw routine sequential coagulation studies, including platelet counts, D-dimer levels, prothrombin time, and partial thromboplastin time. These tests allow clinicians to determine if the clotting cascade has been affected by COVID-19 and whether the patient needs anticoagulation therapy. In severe cases, thrombectomy is a part of the COVID-19 treatment strategy.

Kidney Problems

In addition to the respiratory pathology and coagulopathy, a high percentage of COVID-19 patients are presenting with signs and symptoms of kidney problems. Pei et al. identified that "renal abnormalities occurred in the majority of patients with COVID-19 pneumonia."[26] ICU patients with COVID-19 very often present with this pathology. According to the same study, "Although proteinuria, hematuria, and acute kidney injury (AKI) often resolved within 3 weeks after the onset of symptoms, renal complications in COVID-19 were associated with higher mortality."[26] Microvascular injury and coagulopathy may be significant contributors to renal dysfunction.

For EMS providers, the downstream concerns of kidney problems include electrolyte derangements and hemodynamic fluctuations. The investigators in this study concluded that the patients with acute kidney injury often demonstrated a worse course. It is possible that the microvascular injury and coagulopathy were major contributors to renal dysfunction.

Hospitalizations: Rates and Trends

As the COVID-19 situation evolves, reporting and analysis of hospitalization rates continue to evolve. On June 28, 2020, the CDC reported that the United States had more than 2.5 million cases of COVID-19, with 125,000 deaths. The overall cumulative hospitalization rate was 98.4 per 100,000 population, meaning approximately 0.1% of the country had been hospitalized for COVID-19.[27] It is important to note that hospitalization numbers are

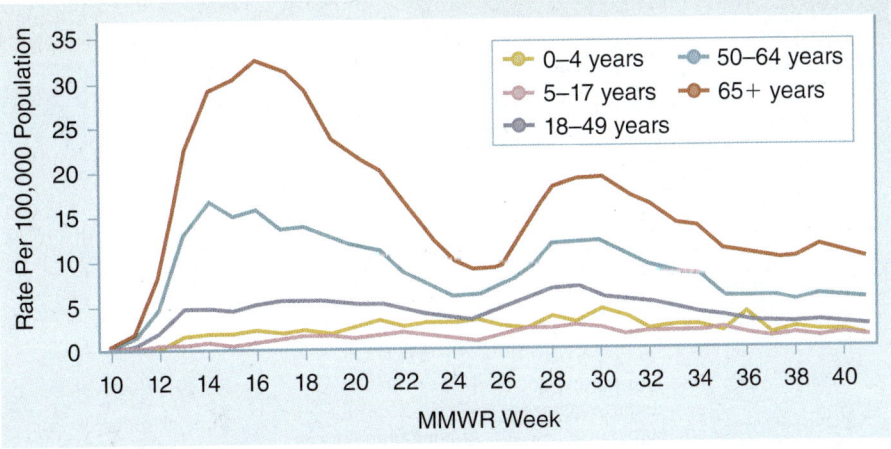

FIGURE 4-4 Hospitalization rates by age group.

Abbreviation: MMWR Week, *Morbidity and Mortality Weekly Report*

From COVID-NET: COVID-19-Associated Hospitalization Surveillance Network, Centers for Disease Control and Prevention. https://gis
.cdc.gov/grasp/COVIDNet/COVID19_5.html. Accessed October 19, 2020.

usually delayed by approximately 2 weeks because they require COVID-NET data from hospitals.

Total hospitalizations have continued to rise in the United States. The highest rate of hospitalization remains among adults aged 65 years or older, followed by adults aged 50 to 64 years, then those aged 18 to 49 years (**FIGURE 4-4**). The total number of deaths has also risen. By October 13, 2020, the CDC reported that the United States had almost 7.8 million cases of COVID-19, with 214,446 deaths.[27]

Drug Development: Highly Targeted and Fast-Tracked

The process of discovering, developing, and eventually manufacturing new medications has changed significantly in recent years. Classic pharmacology looked at the active ingredients of current treatments and tried to line them up with the target disease process. With advances in the use of the human genome, the process today is entirely different, with high throughput screenings against biologic targets.

In the case of SARS-CoV-2, the genome of the virus was mapped and shared in early 2020, enabling the process of drug discovery to be targeted at the different phases and steps in the disease cascade.

In one illness framework, developed by Dr. Salim Rezaie, an emergency medicine physician, the disease process is separated into three phases: viremic, pulmonary, and severe[28] (**TABLE 4-3**).

- During the viremic phase, the viral load of the patient rises sharply, and pharmacology development is being targeted to mitigate viral replication. Antiviral medications work to interrupt that process.

- If the disease progresses to the pulmonary phase, the inflammatory cascade begins to rise sharply. As discussed previously, a dangerous part of the disease process involves an exaggerated inflammatory response and the resulting ARDS and acute kidney injury. Medications focused on blunting the inflammatory response are most effective here. In July 2020, the RECOVERY trial published a set of recommendations regarding dexamethasone during this phase.

- The severe phase has high mortality rates. This phase requires aggressive anti-inflammatory and anticoagulation therapy.

TABLE 4-3 Framework for COVID-19 Phases and Treatment Suggestions

			Time →
Phase	Viremic	Pulmonary	Severe
Immune response	Primarily host viral response	Decreasing viral response, increasing inflammatory response	Primarily host inflammatory response
Drug classifications	Antiviral therapy	Antiviral, corticosteroids, anticoagulants, convalescent plasma	Corticosteroids, anticoagulants, inflammatory inhibitors
Drug effects	Reduces duration of symptoms, minimizes contagiousness, potentially reduces progression of disease	Anti-inflammatory therapy	Anti-inflammatory and immunomodulatory therapy

Based on Rezaie S: The RECOVERY Trial: Dexamethasone for COVID-19? https://rebelem.com/the-recovery-trial-dexamethasone-for-covid-19/. Accessed October 9, 2020.

Trials and Approaches

Development of COVID-19 drugs and therapies continues on several fronts. The FDA created a special coronavirus treatment acceleration program (CTAP) in April 2020 to help get treatments to patients faster.[29] In July, the CTAP dashboard counted more than 570 drugs in the developmental stage and at least 270 trials under review. By August 2020, CTAP displayed 590 drugs in development, 310 trials under review, and 5 drugs approved for emergency use. The August 31, 2020, emergency use authorization (EUA) covers convalescent plasma, remdesivir, and several other emerging therapies[29] (**FIGURE 4-5**).

In May 2020, the National Health Service in the United Kingdom, in collaboration with the University of Birmingham, published a useful global overview of clinical trials[31] (**FIGURE 4-6**). Although other significant studies have emerged since then, this overview helps illustrate the diversity of approaches across the pathologic cascade of events.

With so many treatments and approaches in process, it may be useful to see the clinical picture in terms of treatment types:

- Antivirals, such as remdesivir, lopinavir, and ritonavir, are intended to work by blocking the initial replication of the RNA carried inside the coronavirus.

- Ravulizumab and gemtuzumab ozogamicin work by inhibiting the antibodies and complementary proteins needed in the next step of the cascade.

About Emergency Use Authorization (EUA)

On February 4, 2020, the Secretary of HHS determined that SARS-CoV-2 had the potential to affect national security, and a public health emergency was declared. On March 27, HSS stated, "Circumstances exist justifying the authorization of emergency use of drugs and biological products during the COVID-19 pandemic."[30] This declaration allowed the FDA commissioner to issue EUA for some therapies to be used prior to completing a traditional cycle of trial and peer review when no other adequate therapies existed.

Type of COVID-19 Treatment Being Studied[1]

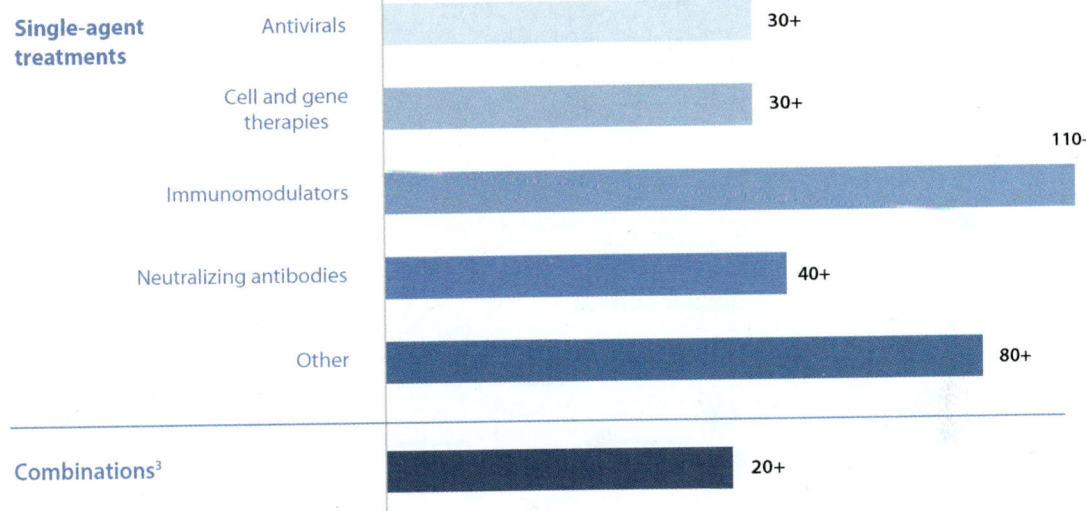

FIGURE 4-5 CTAP dashboard snapshot from August 2020.

[1]Corresponds to number of safe to proceed investigational new drugs (INDs); excludes INDs related to vaccines

[2]For additional information, please see Cellular & Gene Therapy Products

[3]Includes INDs with more than one product

From U.S. Food and Drug Administration. Coronavirus Treatment Acceleration Program (CTAP). https://www.fda.gov/drugs/coronavirus-covid-19
-drugs/coronavirus-treatment-acceleration-program-ctap. Accessed October 15, 2020.

- GSK2798745 and GSK2193874 are channel blockers that decrease the permeability of the endothelial cells in the lungs, which helps reduce pulmonary edema. Similarly, interferon beta 1a and stem cell therapy are also being investigated to help protect against ARDS.

- Azithromycin is a macrolide antibiotic that degranulates, or inhibits the neutrophil response. It is also suggested that it may alter the packaging of the ACE-2 receptor and thus change the initial viral entry into the cell.

- Namilumab inhibits the immune cell proliferation downstream from the alveolar macrophages.

- Dexamethasone is showing promise in inhibiting the cytokine storm.

- Hydroxychloroquine inhibits the B cell activation and thus affects the inflammatory/immune cascade.

- Icatibant, a bradykinin B_2 receptor antagonist, is intended to interrupt the endothelial hyperinflammatory reaction.

Another notable therapy is convalescent plasma. Patients who have recovered from COVID-19 retain some of the antibodies in high enough quantities that they can be beneficial to other patients (**FIGURE 4-7**). A plasma donation from a recovered COVID-19 patient can potentially help up to three additional patients, depending on how soon after the disease donation occurs. This treatment is currently allowable as an investigational treatment under the FDA's EUA program.

Although potentially promising, these treatments are relatively early in their accelerated trials. Researchers are carefully monitoring efficacy, side effects, interactions, and other issues as they advance toward effective treatments.

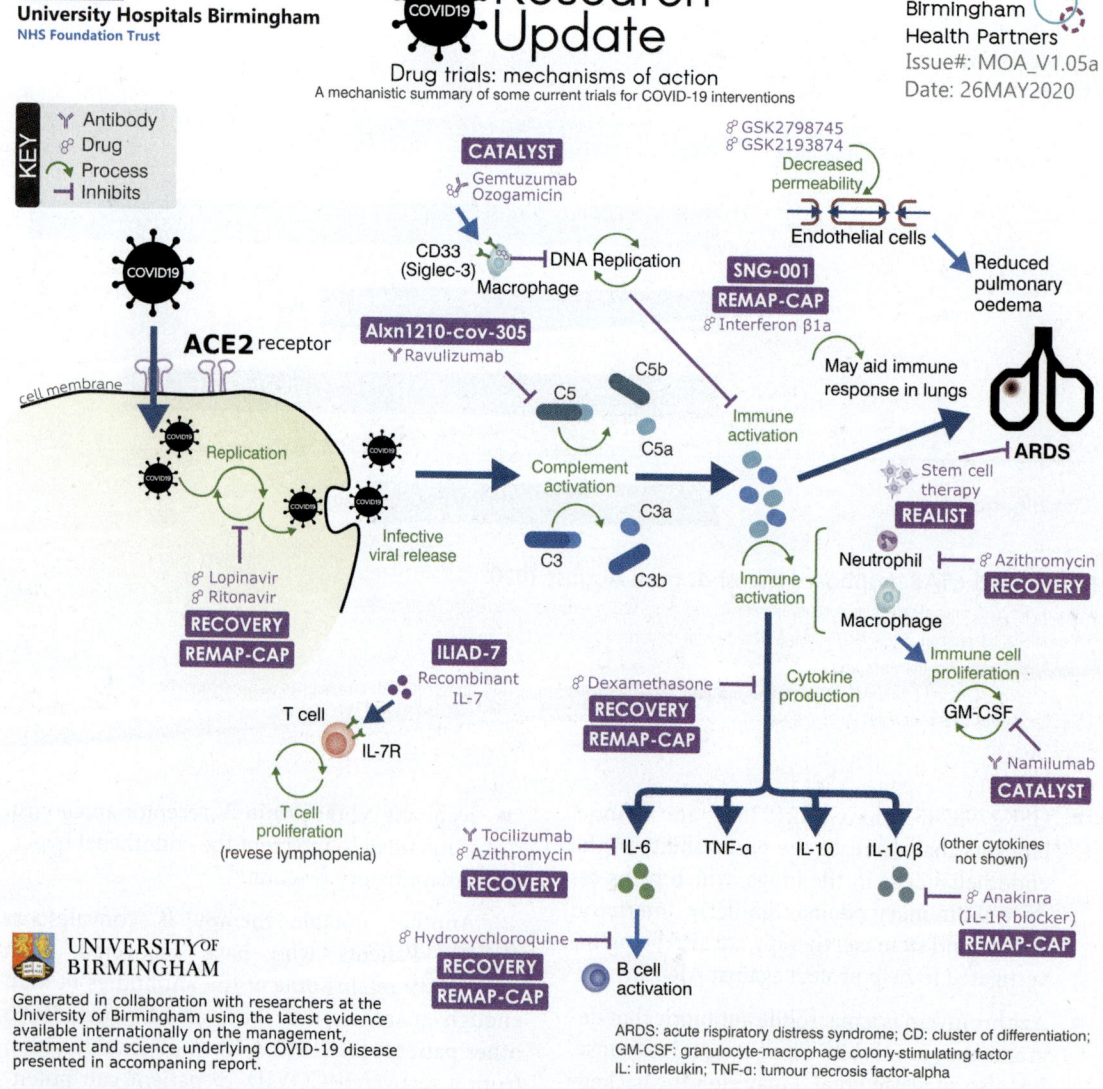

FIGURE 4-6 The worldwide approach to COVID-19 treatment clinical trials.

Used with permission of University of Birmingham.

Considerations for EMS Providers

Most treatments and trials are designed for the in-hospital treatment of patients with COVID-19. Dexamethasone is the only trial medication that is currently available to some prehospital providers. Treatment protocols will be determined by the EMS agency. Oxygen administration combined with strategies such as CPAP can be extremely helpful in managing COVID-19 patients at the scene. Most services that provide CPAP are

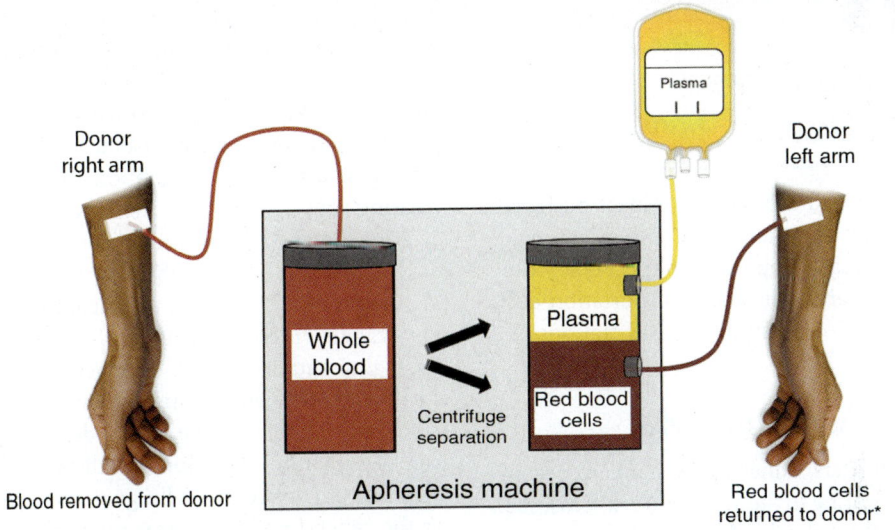

FIGURE 4-7 The convalescent plasma process.

Abbreviation: RBCs, red blood cells

Used wih permission of David H. Spach, MD (University of Washington/IDEA Program: COVID-19 Treatment).

familiar with how to transport and filter the device safely.

Patient safety becomes a major concern when proning is considered during transport. Seat belts and harnesses are not usually designed for prone transport. Also, sudden deterioration would be extremely difficult to manage alone, in the back of a moving ambulance, for a patient being transported in the prone position. When considering the risks and benefits for transport procedures, exercise additional caution regarding prone patients and seek specific guidance from your medical director. The value of short-term proning in the EMS environment has not been clearly established in this or any other population of patients.

The acuity of COVID-19 symptoms remains quite variable, and the challenge is complicated by the fact that some patients may not even know they are infected. Care in the prehospital environment continues to focus on supporting the patient's ventilation and circulation, while minimizing COVID-19 exposure to providers.

PART 5
Public Health Implications

COVID-19 has had a profound impact on health care systems around the world. For EMS providers, the public health implications affect everything from patient interactions and transportation decisions to the basic operation of EMS stations and agencies.

Public Safety and EMS

For EMS providers, adhering to standard recommendations relating to the SARS-CoV-2 virus, such as physical distancing and environmental disinfection, can be extremely challenging. It is recommended that you attempt to maintain a distance of at least 6 feet from others whenever possible, when on duty and off. In addition, discourage large groups from gathering on scene, and limit extra riders in the EMS vehicle whenever possible. Similarly, limiting the number of EMS personnel and other responders on scene or in any crowded or tight spaces can help reduce potential exposures (**FIGURE 5-1**).

Numerous studies have demonstrated the spread of the SARS-CoV-2 virus via both droplets and physical contact. Airborne transmission, particularly in indoor settings with poor ventilation,

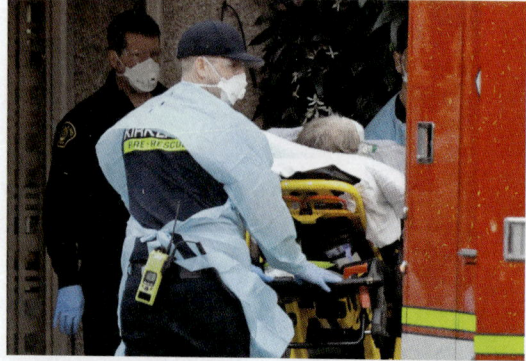

FIGURE 5-1 Distancing for EMS providers is challenging but crucial.
© Ted S. Warren/AP/Shutterstock.

is an increased concern when people congregate indoors due to cooler weather. Models suggest the potential for airborne virus transmission at distances up to 8 meters (approximately 26 to 27 feet), well beyond the current distance recommended for social distancing.[32] Additionally, there is increasing concern that airborne virus spread occurs even in the absence of known aerosol-generating procedures, such as intubation, forceful coughing, bag-mask ventilation, and nebulizer therapy.[5] Physical activities requiring heavy breathing, such as singing and exercising, have been linked to increased airborne virus transmission.

Many EMS and first responder activities inherently require very limited distance between provider and patients, colleagues and coworkers, or the general public. A large portion of these activities require direct physical contact. In addition, EMS providers may be more vulnerable to airborne transmissions emitted during procedures such as open suctioning of airways and cardiopulmonary resuscitation. Approximately 6 months into the COVID-19 pandemic, a small study found the fatality rate for COVID-19 per 100,000 people to be almost 50% higher for EMS providers than for the general population, at 91 per 100,000 versus 62 per 100,000, respectively.[33] Therefore, proper use of the correct PPE is absolutely essential.

Specific precautions and protocols for EMS providers will vary by agency. These measures are crucial to limit transmission risk to providers and the community. They may include changes in patient assessments, efforts to diminish aerosols, and practices to limit the duration or intensity of EMS provider exposure.

An example of a revised practice intended to prevent the transmission of COVID-19 is the use of metered dose inhalers instead of nebulized medications for certain respiratory emergencies. Nebulizers aerosolize medications and are thought to also aerosolize virus particles, releasing them into the environment. If nebulized medications must be used, many organizations advise attempting to administer them in a negative pressure environment, using a nebulizer mask instead of a T-piece and covering it with a surgical/procedural mask. Providers are also advised to perform these procedures on scene whenever possible, avoiding their use in the back of a confined ambulance.[34]

The American Heart Association (AHA) has released revised guidelines for resuscitation of patients who have or are suspected of having COVID-19.[35] These guidelines include the use of filters and a tight seal during bag-mask ventilations. The CDC, AHA, and others advocate for a HEPA-rated filter on bag-mask devices and ventilators to avoid releasing contaminated exhaled ventilation into the environment. Other strategies include use of supraglottic or extraglottic airway devices in lieu of endotracheal intubation, when possible, or having the most experienced provider perform airway procedures to minimize the duration of exposure.

CPAP, PPV, and other respiratory interventions have been shown to produce aerosolized virus particles. EMS providers can expect their organizations to provide guidelines for N95 respirator use and other protective measures applied during these procedures. A variety of sources are also recommending the use of a surgical/procedural mask over an oxygen delivery device, including nonrebreathing masks and high-flow nasal cannulas.

All of these new procedures and guidelines are intended to protect EMS providers and others from exposure to COVID-19. As new research is performed and new lessons are learned, these procedures and guidelines will continue to evolve.

Supporting Testing and Contact Tracing

Testing people for infection with SARS-CoV-2 fulfills a number of public health obligations. A symptomatic person who tests positive may benefit from a number of medications or treatment strategies that may not be indicated for other infectious causes; such strategies include specific antiviral medications, corticosteroids, and other treatment adjuncts.[36] Infection and antibody test results provide an important perspective when making clinical decisions, such as the following:

- Determining clinical treatment strategies
- Assessing the need for isolation precautions
- Determining the necessary PPE

- Considering cohorting patients (keeping those with the same medical condition closer together)

Test results will also affect whether infected people need to isolate or quarantine to protect others. As defined by the CDC, isolation refers to people staying away from others when they *are* infected; quarantine refers to people staying away from others when they *might be* infected.[37]

The CDC recommends a variety of indications and timelines for people with COVID-19 to avoid close contacts, return to work, and receive elective medical care.[38] Given the risk of false-negative results, people with high-risk exposures, travel, or suspicious symptoms may still need to endure a prolonged quarantine to minimize the risk of inadvertently spreading the virus to others despite early negative test results after initial exposure. (**FIGURE 5-2**).

Aggregated test results become extremely important when monitoring the spread or containment of the overall pandemic. Public health, government, and private sector leaders use these data and other key indicators to guide an array of decisions impacting every facet of public life, including the implementation or relaxation of public health orders, the allocation of scarce resources such as PPE or health care personnel, and patient distribution.

Key test-based indicators used to monitor the status of the pandemic include the following:

- Raw total of positive cases
- Positive tests per fixed population (often per 100,000 or 1 million overall population)
- Test positivity rates
- Demographic distribution

Public health officials use a strategy known as contact tracing to slow the spread of COVID-19, as well as other infectious diseases. Contact tracing involves identifying a person who tests positive for the SARS-CoV-2 virus and then identifying other people who have been in contact with that person. Those who have been in contact with the infected person are instructed to monitor for symptoms and quarantine until an adequate amount of time has passed without symptoms (**FIGURE 5-3**).

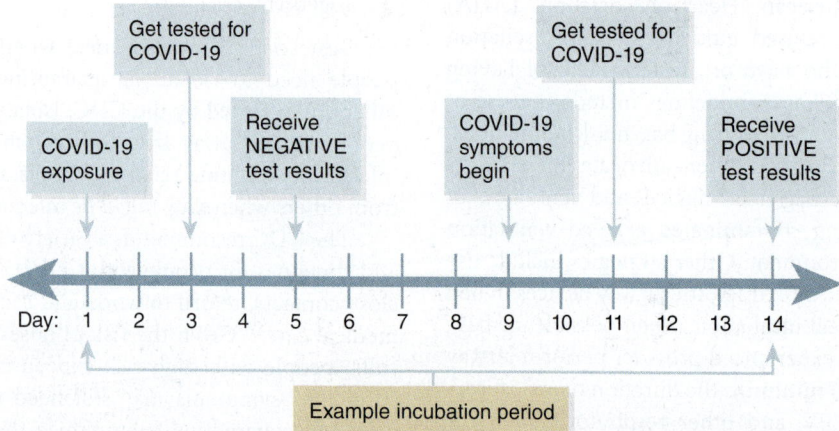

Quarantine for 14 days from your last exposure to someone who has COVID-19.

Get tested for COVID-19

Get tested for COVID-19

COVID-19 exposure

Receive NEGATIVE test results

COVID-19 symptoms begin

Receive POSITIVE test results

Day: 1 2 3 4 5 6 7 8 9 10 11 12 13 14

Example incubation period

• Contraction of COVID-19 can occur any time during the incubation period.
• If exposure occurred at noon on Day 1, quarantine until noon on Day 14.

FIGURE 5-2 Representative isolation and quarantine guidance.

Data from Centers for Disease Control and Prevention: Coronavirus disease 2019 (COVID-19). https://www.cdc.gov/coronavirus/2019-ncov/if-you-are-sick/quarantine.html. Accessed September 10, 2020.

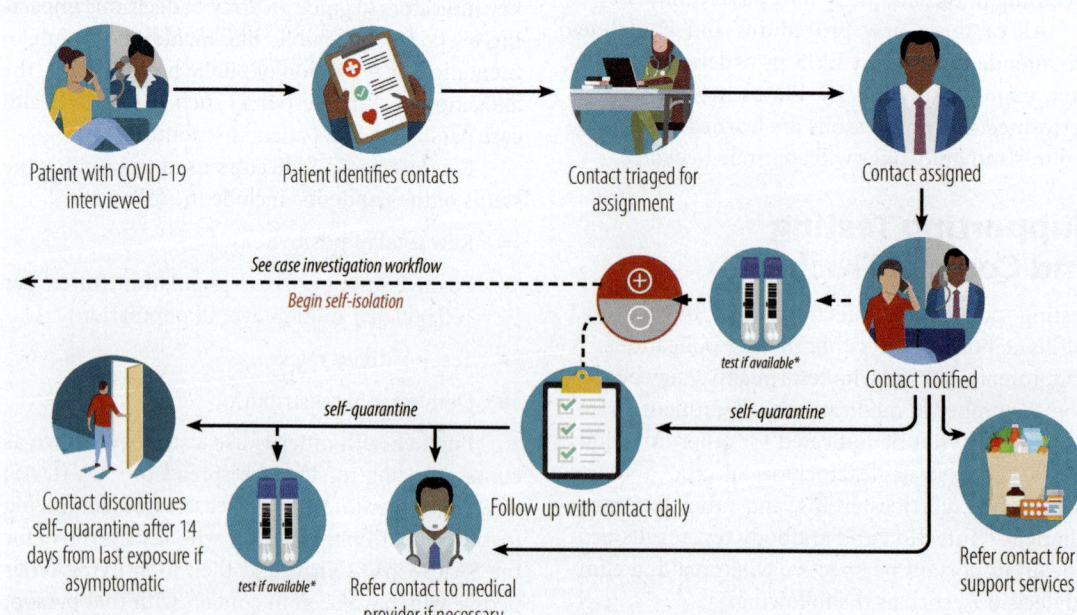

Patient with COVID-19 interviewed

Patient identifies contacts

Contact triaged for assignment

Contact assigned

See case investigation workflow

Begin self-isolation

*test if available**

Contact notified

self-quarantine

self-quarantine

Contact discontinues self-quarantine after 14 days from last exposure if asymptomatic

*test if available**

Follow up with contact daily

Refer contact for support services

Refer contact to medical provider if necessary

FIGURE 5-3 CDC contact tracing guidelines.

* If contact tests positive or develops COVID-19 symptoms, case investigation is necessary.

Reproduced from Centers for Disease Control and Prevention. Contact Tracing for COVID-19. https://www.cdc.gov/coronavirus/2019-ncov/php/contact-tracing/contact-tracing-plan/contact-tracing.html. Accessed September 10, 2020.

Safety Within Congregate Settings

COVID-19 has widely proliferated through many congregate living facilities such as skilled nursing facilities, prisons, and homeless shelters. These facilities face many unique challenges in preventing disease transmission. EMS providers who work in or respond to these settings frequently encounter facilities with PPE shortages, inadequate staffing, rapid transmission of COVID-19 among residents, barriers to prompt virus testing, and additional introduction of infections through staff or visitors.

Health care providers in these settings must carefully balance the risk of personal exposure against the risk of patient cross-contamination, often while working with an extremely limited supply of PPE. The surge in cases, combined with massive demand for PPE amid severe supply chain disruptions, has forced many health care facilities and other congregate living facilities to employ novel practices to protect staff.

Early in the pandemic, when N95 filtering face piece respirators had grown scarce, the CDC and other regulatory agencies provided guidance on extended use, limited reuse, and reprocessing (sometimes referred to as resterilization) of N95 masks[39] (**FIGURE 5-4**). These approaches allow single-use, disposable N95 respirators to be used for multiple patients or multiple wearers, often spanning days, weeks, or longer.

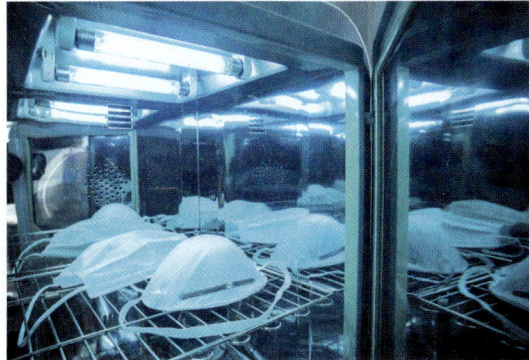

FIGURE 5-4 Resterilizing N95 masks.
© Nor Gal/Shutterstock.

Extended use refers to leaving a mask on through multiple encounters with different patients who are either infected or potentially infected, without removing the mask between encounters. Reuse refers to removing the mask between encounters but using the same mask for multiple patient encounters. Reuse of masks is discouraged when an organism can be spread by contact (fomite) transmission, as the potential for exposure is much higher with repeated donning and doffing.

The FDA has approved a process that uses heated, pressurized hydrogen peroxide to disinfect used N95 respirators without degrading the filter materials for a limited number of times. This system allows for repeated use of the same respirator by multiple wearers without the risk of infectious material remaining on the respirator from one wearer to the next.

EMS and other health care providers working in congregate living facilities may use a combination of single-use disposable PPE and other reuse, extended-use, or reprocessed PPE. A common approach is for the EMS or health care provider to wear the same face piece during the entire work shift, while changing disposable gowns and examination gloves between each patient encounter.

During any PPE removal, it is essential that wearers not contaminate themselves and risk exposure. Many PPE removal procedures require an assistant to safely remove contaminated PPE. Follow your agency's or facility's guidelines, or refer to a reliable source, such as the CDC, for generic instructions for different types of PPE.

Safety in Crew Quarters and Fire Stations

EMS providers in many areas may live in a congregate setting such as a firehouse or EMS station for many consecutive days while on prolonged duty. In this setting, where workers may be seeking rest or a break in a communal area, physical distancing practices can be difficult to follow; however, precautions must be maintained. Consider that each EMS provider, firefighter, or other first responder is at an increased risk for active COVID-19 infection, as discussed previously. These high-risk providers are now cloistered together, where any single provider can infect countless others. Thus, not only might staffing needs in this vital profession be compromised, but the very professionals charged with safeguarding the public might instead spread the disease to high-risk patients.

An alarming number of COVID-19 clusters have developed in fire stations around the United States, prompting specific guidance from the CDC, the US Fire Administration, and various other agencies.[40] Some key recommendations for EMS providers and firefighters living in congregate settings during COVID-19 have emerged (**TABLE 5-1**).

Coping With Health Care Capacity Demands

The massive spread of COVID-19 has pushed many states, regions, and health systems to increase hospital and health care system capacity. EMS providers may see new temporary field hospitals opening as the pandemic continues. The US military has opened at least 17 additional temporary hospital sites, although many have had limited patient care activity. Many other state-based National Guard units have been deployed to a wide variety of COVID-related activities to support field hospitals, health care facilities, and other congregate settings. Hospitals throughout the country have implemented surge plans to increase overall hospital or ICU capacity, including the use of alternate care sites.

As regions or individual hospitals experience a patient surge, they often cancel elective appointments and surgeries to preserve PPE and other resources. They also reposition staff to optimize patient care capabilities when a high patient volume and acuity are present.

All of these efforts have the potential to affect transportation destination choices for EMS providers. EMS providers performing both prehospital

TABLE 5-1 EMS Recommendations for Congregate Living Settings	
✓	Screen all incoming EMS personnel and visitors for fever and other symptoms of COVID-19.
✓	Wear face mask at all times including station breakrooms, etc.
✓	Encourage sick employees to stay home or quarantine as appropriate.
✓	Practice frequent hand hygiene, including readily accessible hand sanitizer dispensers.
✓	Install physical barriers (such as sneeze guards, plexiglass, etc.) between personnel and the general public.
✓	Do not admit or invite nonessential visitors to EMS station, including families.
✓	Maintain physical distance at EMS station or firehouse, especially while eating/drinking or when masks cannot be worn.
✓	Optimize staffing; consider reassignment of nonessential station personnel. Limit comingling and limit larger gatherings.
✓	Provide stress management or peer support services.
✓	Frequently clean and disinfect common areas, bunk rooms, etc.

Data from Centers for Disease Control and Prevention. 2020. *Interim Recommendations for Emergency Medical Services (EMS) Systems and 911 Public Safety Answering Points/Emergency Communication Centers (PSAP/ECCs) in the United States During the Coronavirus Disease (COVID-19) Pandemic.* https://www.cdc.gov/coronavirus/2019-ncov/hcp/guidance-for-ems.html. Accessed November 6, 2020; United States Fire Administration (USFA). 2020. *Information for First Responders on Maintaining Operational Capabilities During a Pandemic.* https://www.usfa.fema.gov/coronavirus/planning_response/. Accessed November 6, 2020.

and interfacility patient transports may experience frequent changes in sending or receiving facilities as alternate care sites or inpatient departments are created, expanded, or relocated due to COVID-19. As transport destination changes continue to occur, EMS providers should expect additional guidelines, protocols, or instructions regarding receiving facilities for patients suspected of having COVID-19.

Home Quarantine for EMS Providers

EMS providers may be instructed to isolate or quarantine at home after testing positive for COVID-19, having a high-risk exposure, or engaging in an activity that creates the risk of virus transmission. EMS regulatory departments and individual EMS agencies may have specific protocols for personnel to follow while under isolation or quarantine (**TABLE 5-2**).

Maintaining Perspective: Now and in the Future

COVID-19 has dramatically changed many facets of public life, including the ways in which EMS providers interact with patients, each other, and their workplace. It is impossible to predict how long these changes will last or what practices will remain indefinitely. It is certainly possible that the COVID-19 pandemic will make certain public health measures, such as wearing a mask, a permanent part of our lives, just as mask wearing has become routine in parts of eastern Asia.

The public health implications of this pandemic will continue to have a significant impact on the EMS profession. As professionals on the front lines, it is vital to follow recommended guidelines and protocols, approach each interaction with care, and stay informed of both agency and public health recommendations as the situation continues to evolve.

TABLE 5-2 Recommended Leave at Home Protocols

LEAVE AT HOME INSTRUCTIONS
Respiratory Infection/Suspected or Confirmed COVID-19

These instructions are for individuals with an acute respiratory infection that are confirmed or suspected to be COVID-19 and do not require hospitalization or emergent care.

✓	Limit contact with household members, any high-risk (susceptible) individuals, and the general public.
✓	Frequently screen for fever or other COVID-19 symptoms, such as loss of taste/smell, respiratory distress, cough, etc.
✓	Do not share personal items such as toothbrush, utensils, towels, etc.
✓	Wash hands frequently.
✓	Wear a mask when in proximity to others.
✓	Plan for follow-up health care if symptoms develop/worsen.
✓	Frequently clean/disinfect common surfaces (doorknobs, handles, remotes, etc.).
✓	Consult your agency or jurisdiction for specific durations of isolation or quarantine, triggers to return to work, and other guidelines.

Data from Whatcom County, Washington, Emergency Medical Services. 2020. *Leave at Home Instructions.* https://naemsp.org/NAEMSP /media/COVID-19-Sample-Protocols/LEAVE-AT-HOME-INSTRUCTIONS-COVID19.pdf. October 12, 2020.

References

1. Burrell CJ: *Fenner and White's Medical Virology.* 5th ed. London, England: Academic Press; 2017.

2. Korsman SNJ: *Virology.* London, England: Churchill Livingstone; 2012.

3. Haagmans B: *Vaccines for Biodefense and Emerging and Neglected Diseases.* London, England: Academic Press; 2009.

4. Information about Middle East respiratory syndrome. Centers for Disease Control and Prevention website. https://www.cdc.gov /coronavirus/mers/downloads /factsheet-mers_en.pdf. Accessed October 6, 2020.

5. Wilson N, Corbett S, Tovey E: Airborne transmission of COVID-19. *The British Medical Journal.* https:// www.bmj.com/content/370/bmj .m3206. Accessed October 6, 2020.

6. Coronavirus (COVID-19) update: Serological tests. US Food and Drug Administration website. https:// www.fda.gov/news-events/press -announcements/coronavirus -covid-19-update-serological-tests. Updated April 7, 2020. Accessed October 6, 2020.

7. Gousseff M, Penot P, Gallay L, et al: Clinical recurrences of COVID-19 symptoms after recovery: Viral relapse, reinfection or inflammatory rebound? *Journal of Infection.* 2020. https://www.ncbi.nlm.nih.gov/pmc /articles/PMC7326402/. Accessed October 6, 2020.

8. Walsh KA, Jordan K, Clyne B, et al: SARS-CoV-2 detection, viral load and infectivity over the course of an infection. *J Infect* 2020;81(3):357-371.

9. van Doremale, Neeltje, Trenton Bushmaker, Dylan H. Morris, et al: Aerosol and surface stability of SARS-CoV-2 as compared with SARS-CoV-1. *N Engl J Med* 2020;382(16):1564-1567.

10. Draft landscape of COVID-19 candidate vaccines. World Health Organization website. https://www .who.int/publications/m/item /draft-landscape-of-covid-19 -candidate-vaccines. Updated October 19, 2020. Accessed October 13, 2020.

11. The journey of your child's vaccine. Centers for Disease Control and Prevention website. www.cdc .gov/vaccines/parents/infographics /journey-of-child-vaccine.html ?CDC_AA_refVal=www.cdc.gov /vaccines/parents/infographics /journey-of-child-vaccine-text .html. January 26, 2018. Accessed October 13, 2020.

12. Wee S-L, Simões M: In coronavirus vaccine race, China strays from the official paths. *The New York Times.* www.nytimes.com/2020/07/16 /business/china-vaccine -coronavirus.html. Updated July 16, 2020. Accessed October 13, 2020.

13. Callaway E: Russia's fast-track coronavirus vaccine draws outrage over safety. *Nature.* https://www.nature .com/articles/d41586-020-02386-2. Updated August 11, 2020. Accessed October 13, 2020.

14. O'Keefe SM: One in three Americans would not get COVID-19 vaccine. Gallup. https://news.gallup .com/poll/317018/one-three -americans-not-covid-vaccine.aspx. Updated August 7, 2020. Accessed October 13, 2020.

15. US Department of Health and Human Services. Fact sheet: Explaining operation warp speed. www.hhs .gov/about/news/2020/06/16 /fact-sheet-explaining-operation -warp-speed.html. September 4, 2020. Accessed October 13, 2020.

16. Malcom K: The top 5 COVID-19 vaccine candidates explained. University of Michigan. labblog.uofmhealth.org/rounds /top-5-covid-19-vaccine -candidates-explained. Updated August 7, 2020. Accessed October 13, 2020.

17. O'Callaghan KP, Blatz AM, Offit PA: Developing a SARS-CoV-2 vaccine at warp speed. *JAMA.* 2020;324(5):437-438.

18. Coppo A, Bellani G, Winterton D, et al: Feasibility and physiological effects of prone positioning in non-intubated patients with acute respiratory failure due to COVID-19 (PRON-COVID): A prospective cohort study. *Lancet Respir Med* 2020;8(8):765-774. https://www.thelancet.com/journals /lanres/article/PIIS2213-2600(20) 30268-X/fulltext.

19. Heneghan C, Pluddemann A, Mahtani KR: Differentiating viral from bacterial pneumonia. Centre for Evidence-Based Medicine website. https://www.cebm.net/covid-19 /differentiating-viral-from -bacterial-pneumonia/. Updated April 8, 2020. Accessed October 13, 2020.

20. Burk M, El Kersh K, Saad M, Wiemken T, Ramirez J, Cavallazzi R: Viral infection in community-acquired pneumonia: A systematic review and meta-analysis. *Eur Respir Rev* 2016;25:178-188.

21. Caputo N, Strayer RJ, Levitan R: Early self-proning in awake, non-intubated patients in the emergency department: A single ED's experience during the COVID-19 pandemic. *Acad Emerg Med* 2020;27(5):375-378.

22. Salehi S, Abedi A, Balakrishnan S, Gholamresanezhad A: Coronavirus disease 2019 (COVID-19): A systematic review of imaging findings in 919 patients. *AJR Am J Roentgenol* 2020;215(1):87-93.

23. Ye Q, Wang B, Mao J: The pathogenesis and treatment of the 'Cytokine Storm' in COVID-19. *J Infect* 2020;80(6):607-613.

24. Cummings MJ, Baldwin MR, Abrams D, et al: Epidemiology, clinical course, and outcomes of critically ill adults with COVID-19 in New York City: A prospective cohort study. *Lancet* 2020;395(10239):1763 1770.

25. Iba T, Levy JH, Levi M, Connors JM, Thachil J: Coagulopathy of coronavirus disease 2019. *Crit Care Med* 2020; 48(9):1358-1364.

26. Pei G, Zhang Z, Peng J, et al: Renal involvement and early prognosis in patients with COVID-19 pneumonia. *J Am Soc Nephrol* 2020;31(6):1157-1165.

27. COVID view: A weekly surveillance summary of US COVID-19 activity. Centers for Disease Control and Prevention website. https://www .cdc.gov/coronavirus/2019-ncov /covid-data/covidview/index.html. Updated October 9, 2020. Accessed October 13, 2020.

28. Rezaie S: The RECOVERY trial: Dexamethasone for COVID-19? REBELEM website. https:// rebelem.com/the-recovery-trial -dexamethasone-for-covid-19/. Updated June 23, 2020. Accessed October 13, 2020.

29. Coronavirus treatment acceleration program (CTAP). US Food and Drug Administration website. https://www.fda.gov/drugs /coronavirus-covid-19-drugs /coronavirus-treatment -acceleration-program-ctap. Updated September 30, 2020. Accessed October 13, 2020.

30. US Department of Health and Human Services. Emergency use authorization declaration. Federal Register. https://www.federalregister .gov/documents/2020/04/01/2020 -06905/emergency-use -authorization-declaration. Accessed October 13, 2020.

31. COVID-19 research briefing. University of Birmingham website. https://www.birmingham.ac.uk /university/colleges/mds /Coronavirus/COVID-19-research -briefing.aspx. Accessed October 13, 2020.

32. Klompas M, Baker MA, Rhee C: Airborne transmission of SARS-CoV-2: Theoretical considerations and available evidence. *JAMA* 2020;324(5):441-442.

33. Maguire BJ, O'Neill BJ, Phelps S, Maniscalco PM, Gerard DR, Handal KA: COVID-19 fatalities among EMS clinicians. EMS1. https://www .ems1.com/ems-products/personal -protective-equipment-ppe/articles /covid-19-fatalities-among-ems -clinicians-BMzHbuegIn1xNLrP/. Accessed October 13, 2020.

34. Indiana Department of Homeland Security. *Indiana Department of Homeland Security COVID-19 EMS Manual.* https://www.in.gov /dhs/files/IDHS-COVID-19 -Manual-04162020.pdf. Accessed October 13, 2020.

35. BLS healthcare provider adult cardiac arrest algorithm for suspected or confirmed COVID-19 patients. American Heart Association website. https://cpr.heart.org/-/media /cpr-files/resources/covid-19 -resources-for-cpr-training/english /algorithmbls_adult_cacovid _200406.pdf?la=en. Updated April 2020. Accessed October 13, 2020.

36. Corum J, Wu KJ, Zimmer C: Coronavirus drug and treatment tracker. *The New York Times.* https://www .nytimes.com/interactive/2020 /science/coronavirus-drugs -treatments.html. Updated October 4, 2020. Accessed October 13, 2020.

37. When to quarantine. Centers for Disease Control and Prevention website. https://www.cdc.gov /coronavirus/2019-ncov/if-you-are -sick/quarantine.html?CDC_AA _refVal=https%3A%2F%2Fwww .cdc.gov%2Fcoronavirus%2F2019 -ncov%2Fif-you-are-sick%2 Fquarantine-isolation.html. Updated September 10, 2020. Accessed October 13, 2020.

38. How to protect yourself and others. Centers for Disease Control and Prevention website. https://www .cdc.gov/coronavirus/2019-ncov /prevent-getting-sick/prevention .html. Updated September 11, 2020. Accessed October 13, 2020.

39. Pandemic planning. Centers for Disease Control and Prevention website. https://www.cdc.gov/niosh /topics/hcwcontrols/recommended guidanceextuse.html. Updated March 27, 2020. Accessed October 13, 2020.

40. Interim recommendations for Emergency Medical Services (EMS) Systems and 911 Public Safety Answering Points/Emergency Communication Centers (PSAP/ECCs) in the United States during the coronavirus disease (COVID-19) pandemic. Centers for Disease Control and Prevention website. https:// www.cdc.gov/coronavirus/2019 -ncov/hcp/guidance-for-ems.html. Updated July 15, 2020. Accessed October 12, 2020.

Additional Resources

All Things Considered. US field hospitals stand down, most without treating any COVID-19 patients. National Public Radio. https://www.npr.org/2020/05/07/851712311/u-s-field-hospitals-stand-down-most-without-treating-any-covid-19-patients. May 7, 2020. Accessed October 13, 2020.

American Hospital Association. Coronavirus update: Technology for the decontamination and reuse of N95 respirators now available. https://www.aha.org/advisory/2020-04-08-coronavirus-update-technology-decontamination-and-reuse-n95-respirators-now. Accessed October 13, 2020.

American Thoracic Society. Top 20 pneumonia facts—2019. https://www.thoracic.org/patients/patient-resources/resources/top-pneumonia-facts.pdf. Accessed October 13, 2020.

Argyropoulos KV, Serrano A, Hu J, et al: Association of initial viral load in severe acute respiratory syndrome coronavirus 2 (SARS-CoV-2) patients with outcome and symptoms. *A J Pathol* 2020;190(9):1881-1887.

Calfee CS, Delucchi K, Parsons PE, et al: Subphenotypes in acute respiratory distress syndrome: Latent class analysis of data from two randomised controlled rrials. *Lancet Respir Med* 2014;2(8):611-620.

Carpenter CR, Mudd PA, West CP, et al: Diagnosing COVID-19 in the emergency department: A scoping review of clinical examinations, laboratory tests, imaging accuracy, and biases. *Acad Emerg Med* 2020. June 16;10.1111/acem.14048.

Centers for Disease Control and Prevention. 2019–2020 US flu season: Preliminary in-season burden estimates. https://www.cdc.gov/flu/about/burden/preliminary-in-season-estimates.htm. Updated October 1, 2020. Accessed October 6, 2020.

Centers for Disease Control and Prevention. Clinical questions about COVID-19: Questions and answers. https://www.cdc.gov/coronavirus/2019-ncov/hcp/faq.html#Infection-Control. Updated August 4, 2020. Accessed October 13, 2020.

Centers for Disease Control and Prevention. How COVID-19 spreads. https://www.cdc.gov/coronavirus/2019-ncov/prevent-getting-sick/how-covid-spreads.html. Updated October 5, 2020. Accessed October 13, 2020.

Centers for Disease Control and Prevention. Human coronavirus types. https://www.cdc.gov/coronavirus/types.html#:~:text=People%20around%20the%20world%20commonly,and%20MERS%2DCoV. Updated February 5, 2020. Accessed October 6, 2020.

Famous KR, Delucchi K, Ware LB, et al: Acute respiratory distress syndrome subphenotypes respond differently to randomized fluid management strategy. *Am J Respir Crit Care Med* 2017;195(3):331-338.

Fu Z, Tang N, Chen Y, Ma L: CT features of COVID-19 patients with two consecutive negative RT-PCR tests after treatment. *Sci Rep* 2020;10(1):11548.

Harvard Medical School. COVID-19 basics. https://www.health.harvard.edu/diseases-and-conditions/covid-19-basics. Accessed October 13, 2020.

Infectious Diseases Education and Assessment. Convalescent plasma. https://covid.idea.medicine.uw.edu/page/treatment/drugs/human-coronavirus-immune-plasma-hcip. Accessed October 13, 2020.

Johns Hopkins University of Medicine. Daily state-by-state testing trends. https://coronavirus.jhu.edu/testing/individual-states. Accessed October 13, 2020.

Li J, Fink JB, Ehrmann S: High-flow nasal cannula for COVID-19 patients: Low risk of bio-aerosol dispersion. *Eur Respir J* 2020;55(5):2000892.

Roche JA, Roche R: A hypothesized role for dysregulated bradykinin signaling in COVID-19 respiratory complications. *FASEB J* 2020;34(6):7265-7269.

Setti L, Passarini F, De Gennaro G, et al: Airborne transmission route of COVID-19: Why 2 meters/6 feet of inter-personal distance could not be enough. *Int J Environ Res Public Health* 2020;17(8):2932.

Yuen K-S, Ye Z-W, Fung S-Y, Chan C-P, Jin D-Y: SARS-CoV-2 and COVID-19: The most important research questions. *Cell Biosci* 2020;10(40).